Natural Remedies for Essential Tremor

Natural Remedies for Essential Tremor

Donna M. Gagnon, ND, CNC

The use of information in this book is intended to be for educational purposes only. It is not intended to be a substitute for professional medical advice, diagnosis, or treatment. If you have symptoms or suffer from an illness, consult with an appropriate healthcare practitioner before carrying out any information presented in this book. Any changes to diet, medications, nutritional supplements, or exercise patterns should be approved and monitored by your physician or other healthcare practitioner.

LoriRay Publishing
P.O. Box 34291
Reno, Nevada 89533

ISBN-13: 9780692495926
ISBN-10: 0692495924
Library of Congress Control Number: 2015947735
LoriRay Publishing, Reno, NV

Table of Contents

Introduction

Essential Tremor (ET) is one of the most common afflictions, affecting about 1 percent of people in the world. Yet it is often misdiagnosed, leading to improper drug treatments. Researchers have not found a cure—meaning that no conventional treatment today has been found to eliminate the symptoms completely. There is no medication made specifically for ET. High blood pressure, anxiety, and seizure medications have produced mixed results for ET patients. Surgery is available with varying outcomes and degrees of risk.

When symptoms first appear, a patient with ET usually goes to a doctor—whose first line of defense is to write a prescription. If the first drug doesn't work, another is tried. Doctors rarely use natural methods of healing because they do not receive adequate training in nutrition or healthy lifestyle choices in medical school. This is unfortunate, since drugs often cover up symptoms, never getting to the root of the problem. Drugs can also have risky side effects. Natural methods, in addition to their healing effects, may work just as well or better than prescription drugs, usually with fewer side effects and less expense.

Most people with ET do not know what causes their symptoms. This doesn't mean there is no cause. It may be exposure to an environmental toxin, a nutritional deficiency, a side effect of a prescription drug, a low-functioning thyroid, or solely genetic. It may also be a combination of things. Unless your doctor asks you the right questions and performs the right diagnostic tests, he or she may miss important clues. This book will point you in the right direction and help you find the reason or reasons for your tremors. Even if you do not uncover a specific cause for them, you will discover an abundance of information on what can trigger tremors or make them worse.

People with symptoms of chronic shaking from any cause have a central nervous system (CNS) dysfunction. The CNS comprises the brain and the spinal cord. The brain plays a central role in the control of most bodily functions, including awareness, thoughts, memory, movements, sensations, and speech. The spinal cord is connected to the brain stem. Nerves exit the spinal cord to both sides of the body. The spinal cord carries signals or messages back and forth between the brain and the peripheral nerves. Therefore, if the brain, nerves, and/or spinal cord are not functioning properly, any number of symptoms related to CNS dysfunction, such as headaches, muscle weakness, seizures, and *tremors*, can occur. So, healing those areas is critical for the shaking to slow down or cease altogether. All remedies in this book work to heal the brain, nerves, and spinal cord. The degree of improvement you experience with natural treatments depends on several factors: what triggered your tremors, how long you've had them, the severity of your symptoms, your genetics, and your current state of health. Someone with mild tremors who is in fairly good health will likely improve quicker than someone who has severe tremors and is in poor health. In addition, the more natural remedies you follow, the greater your chance of success in a shorter amount of time. Natural remedies do not work like drugs or surgery; they are not a quick fix. Your tremors likely took months or years to develop, so it may take many months to see any significant improvement.

The natural remedies and recommendations in this book also offer the benefit of added protection against other neurodegenerative conditions such as Alzheimer's, Lou Gehrig's disease (ALS), dementia, and multiple sclerosis (MS) as well as cancer, depression, diabetes, heart disease, and weight gain. You will be calmer and healthier. So, join me on this journey of healing. You have nothing to lose and only your health to gain.

Parts I and II provide background information on ET for those who have little knowledge of the condition. Part I includes a discussion on types of tremors, possible causes, risk factors for developing ET, common symptoms, and how ET is diagnosed. Part II includes discussions on pre-scription drugs, surgery, and other current treatment options.

Part III contains detailed descriptions of 24 natural remedies for ET; it is the *raison d'être* for this book.

Part IV helps you design your own personal action plan with a step-by-step approach. First, you will answer a questionnaire that was devised to determine the causes or triggers for your tremors. Then, based on your answers, you will be able to determine which medical tests you should take and which natural remedies will work best for reducing your tremors.

Part I

Overview

1

Tremors Defined

THERE ARE MORE than 20 types of tremor disorders, several with symptoms that overlap. An estimated 30 to 50 percent of essential tremor (ET) diagnoses are incorrect.[1] It is important to understand the differences to ensure that you are diagnosed and treated for the correct one. The most common tremor types are described below.

Parkinsonian Tremor

The cause of Parkinson's disease (PD) is the progressive deterioration of neurons in the area of the brain called the substantia nigra. When functioning normally, these neurons produce a vital brain chemical known as dopamine. A lack of dopamine results in abnormal nerve functioning, causing a loss in the ability to control body movements. Why this deterioration happens is not clear. According to the Parkinson's Disease Foundation, about 15 to 25 percent of people with PD have a relative with it. Several gene mutations can cause the disease, but this accounts for only a small percentage of cases. PD has also been linked to environmental toxins such as manganese, pesticide exposure, and contaminants in well water.[2]

Named for the disease it accompanies, Parkinsonian tremor is caused by damage to structures within the brain that control movement. The tremor is defined as a resting tremor because movement occurs when the muscles of the hands are relaxed and at rest. Resting tremor is usually the first symptom of Parkinson's. It mostly affects the hands but can also affect the chin, lips, legs, and trunk. Stress and emotions can significantly increase tremors.[3]

Available conventional treatment options for Parkinsonian tremor include drugs and surgery. Common drugs include Levodopa and dopamine agonists, anticholinergics, and beta-blockers. Levodopa and dopamine agonists alleviate Parkinsonian tremor in some patients, but often, control is not satisfactory, and side effects can be worse than the original symptoms. Anticholinergics and beta-blockers can reduce tremors, but they also have problematic side effects. Common surgeries include deep brain stimulation (DBS) and thalamotomy.

Cerebellar Tremor (CT)
Cerebellar tremor is caused by lesions or damage to the cerebellum usually resulting from stroke, tumor, traumatic brain injury, and neurodegenerative diseases such as multiple sclerosis (MS). CT is also called "intention tremor" due to the slow shaking of the extremities that occurs at the end of a deliberate movement such as pressing a button. The tremor is often most prominent when the affected person is active or is maintaining a specific posture. CT may be accompanied by speech problems, rapid involuntary movements of the eyes, gait problems, and postural tremor of the trunk and neck.[4]

CT is difficult to treat with medication; however, those that relax the CNS can be helpful. Surgery such as DBS and thalamotomy are other options.

Dystonic Tremor
Dystonic tremor, a symptom of dystonia, is a movement disorder in which a person experiences muscle contractions that cause abnormal movements and unusual postures. Dystonia can affect any part of the body,

including the eyes, neck, arms, and legs. Dystonic tremor occurs irregularly and often can be relieved by complete rest. Touching the affected muscle or body part may reduce tremor intensity.[5] Dystonia and ET have been strongly associated for more than a century. Misdiagnosis is common because mild dystonia is frequently overlooked in patients with ET.

There are three main types of dystonia: acquired, genetic, and idiopathic. Acquired (also called secondary) dystonia is caused by damage to the basal ganglia, the area of the brain that is responsible for initiating muscle contractions. The damage could be the result of brain trauma, drug reactions, infection, oxygen deprivation, poisoning caused by lead or carbon monoxide, stroke, and tumor. Genetic (also called familial or primary) dystonia is inherited from a parent who carries a defective gene. Some carriers of the disorder may never develop dystonia themselves. Symptoms may vary widely among members of the same family. Idiopathic dystonia means the condition developed spontaneously or from an unknown cause.[6]

In this case, medications can help reduce symptoms. Drugs include levodopa, trihexyphenidyl, benztropine, tetrabenazine, diazepam, lorazepam, clonazepam, and baclofen. A recently introduced treatment is botulinum toxin, also called Botox. The toxin is injected into the affected muscle to reduce contractions and improve abnormal postures. Injections must be repeated about every three months.[7]

When dystonia is so severe that it causes disability, deep brain stimulation (DBS) and selective denervation (SD) are other options. SD is a surgical operation used for treating neck dystonia; the nerves that control the overactive muscles responsible for the symptoms are cut.[8]

Orthostatic Tremor (OT)

Orthostatic tremor is characterized by rhythmic muscle contractions that occur in the legs and trunk immediately after standing. The person typically perceives OT as unsteadiness rather than actual tremor. OT is a high-frequency tremor, which means its rhythm is very rapid, with as many as 16 to 20 tremor cycles per second. That's significantly faster than other tremor types. For example, the tremors of ET and Parkinson's disease usually occur at a rate of 8 to 12 and 4 to 8 tremor cycles per second, respectively.[9]

Because the tremor is so fast, OT can be difficult to see, making a diagnosis challenging. When patients report that they feel unsteady on their feet, physicians may overlook the leg tremor and pursue other possible causes of unsteadiness. To check for OT, a doctor can place a hand on the thigh to feel for the tremor or use a stethoscope to hear it.[10]

At the Mayo Clinic, suspected OT can be confirmed by assessing the electrical activity in the leg muscles. In this tremor, the leg muscles show no electrical activity when a person is sitting, but when he or she stands up, the muscles immediately fire rhythmic bursts of electrical activity.[11]

OT can make daily activities that require standing without support difficult or impossible, such as standing in line at a store or at the kitchen counter to prepare a meal. Although most people don't fall as a result of this condition, approximately 15 percent become so unsteady that falling is a problem. However, tremors often stop when a person sits or lies down, and they also decrease during walking.[12]

Although OT tends not to be a progressive disorder, it is often persistent and is unlikely to resolve on its own. Because the cause of OT is unknown, treatment focuses on the symptoms. The first line of treatment is clonazepam or a related drug. This medication works moderately to significantly for about one-third of people with the condition, and for some, it eliminates OT almost entirely.[13]

Psychogenic Tremor

Also called functional tremor, psychogenic tremor can appear as any form of tremor movement and is usually caused by an underlying psychological condition called conversion disorder, a condition in which psychological stress manifests in physical ways. Most psychogenic movement is involuntary and can involve any part of the body. It can resemble the same muscle movements that occur with a biological condition or structural abnormality. But, unlike movement disorders caused by biological or structural conditions, the characteristics of this kind of tremor usually develop suddenly, progress quickly, and come and go with partial or complete remission. Symptoms can greatly decrease or disappear when the individual is distracted. In addition, the course of the condition may be short-lived or lead to chronic disability.[14]

Psychogenic tremor is difficult to diagnose because it mimics many other types of tremors. Treatment typically includes a combination of psychotherapy, placebo, medication for symptoms of depression or anxiety, and physical therapy. People who are younger and those with a shorter duration of symptoms have a better prognosis than older patients and those with chronic symptoms.[15]

Physiologic Tremor

Not considered a neurological disorder, physiologic tremor occurs in every normal individual at some point in life. Physiologic tremor is rarely visible to the eye but can be seen momentarily in the hands when the fingers are fully extended. It is heightened by reaction to triggers, including alcohol withdrawal, caffeine, certain drugs, low blood sugar, an overactive thyroid, physical exhaustion, stimulants, or strong emotion such as anxiety or fear. The tremor usually disappears when the underlying cause is eliminated.

Essential Tremor (ET or Tremor)

Essential tremor is the main type of tremor that this book focuses on. In the late 1800s, physicians recognized a common condition in which abnormal tremors occurred primarily in the upper limbs. In the absence of other neurological signs, they called this condition essential tremor.

ET is the most common tremor disorder except for physiologic tremor, which, for all intents and purposes, is not considered a disorder. It affects men and women equally and can develop at any age, even in children and newborns. Children of a parent who has ET have a 50 percent chance of inheriting the condition. According to the International

Essential Tremor Foundation (IETF), there are approximately 10 million Americans who have ET, most over the age of 40. That is eight times as many as those affected by Parkinson's. But due to celebrity spokespersons like Michael J. Fox and Muhammad Ali, symptoms related to PD have much more visibility in the media than ET, and therefore its research receives much more funding.

The shaking in ET is often confused with that of PD, resulting in many misdiagnoses. In addition, approximately 20 percent of those with ET go on to develop PD. The risk of developing PD has been found to be 4.3 times higher in those with ET than in age-matched controls without ET.[16]

In some, the symptoms of ET may be mild and nonprogressive, while in others, ET progresses slowly but continually. Tremor frequency may decrease with age, but the severity may increase. The hands are most often affected, but the head, voice, tongue, legs, and trunk may also be involved, typically to a lesser extent than the hands. Tremor of the hands is usually present as an action tremor characterized by small, rapid movements. Some people feel an internal tremor. Although rare, the legs and feet can also be affected. Some may experience mild gait disturbances. Many factors may trigger tremors and/or increase their severity, including extreme fatigue, fever, low blood sugar, and stress. ET symptoms are discussed in more detail in Part I, chapter 3.

According to the IETF, few prescription medications are available to relieve the symptoms of ET. Unfortunately, medications are ineffective for an estimated more than 40 percent of patients. Surgery is an option in severe cases and for those in whom medication fails.

People with ET may have trouble holding or using small objects such as silverware or writing utensils. This makes eating, writing, buttoning a shirt, or lifting a glass of water difficult. Those with ET whose careers depend on the use of the hands and arms, such as painting or typing at a computer, are most affected. Because ET affects quality of life, many become embarrassed and self-conscious, which frequently leads to depression and low self-esteem. This makes ET not just a physical condition but a psychological one as well. To be most effective, a treatment plan should consider both conditions.

2

Possible Causes and Risks

ACCORDING TO THE International Essential Tremor Foundation, there is evidence that ET runs in families and is hereditary in more than 50 percent of cases. Each child of a parent who has ET has a 50 percent chance of inheriting a gene that causes the condition. Variants of the genes LINGO1 and LINGO2 have been associated with increased risk of ET, although not all individuals with ET carry these variants.[1] LINGO1 and LINGO2 have also been associated with Parkinson's disease (PD), which links ET to PD. The gene variants can also be present in people without ET.

When more than one member of a family has ET, it is referred to as "familial essential tremor." Familial ET often starts in early middle age, but it may be seen in people who are older or younger. Nothing can be done about family history; however, it may be possible to delay the onset of symptoms or lessen their severity by eliminating or reducing the factors that can trigger or worsen them. Besides family history, researchers have found the following as other risk factors that may increase the odds of developing ET:

Decrease in GABA receptors

The function of the neurotransmitter GABA (gamma-aminobutyric acid) is to reduce the activity of the neurons to which it binds. Some researchers believe that one of the purposes GABA serves is to control the fear or anxiety we experience when neurons are overexcited. Scientists at the Université Laval in Canada found those with ET to have decreased GABA receptor concentrations in the cerebellum, a part of the brain that controls movement and balance. More studies are needed, but researchers believe that such a decrease may contribute to ET symptoms.[2]

Cerebellar degeneration

Some research suggests that the cerebellum does not work correctly in people with ET due to a mild degeneration or dysfunction of certain parts of the cerebellum.[3] This may suggest that ET is linked to CT (intention tremor). More studies are needed.

Medications

Taking certain medications can increase risk of developing ET or worsen existing tremors. Drugs that may cause tremors include (but are not limited to) amphetamines, corticosteroids, and psychotics. Stopping the drug may alleviate the tremors, but this depends on the drug and how long it has been taken. The longer certain drugs are taken, the greater the chance of tremors becoming permanent.

Medical conditions

Common medical conditions that can induce shaking include hyperthyroidism (overactive thyroid) and low estrogen levels. Less common medical conditions that can cause shaking include adrenal-gland dysfunction and liver failure. Liver failure is a critical and life-threatening condition that needs immediate treatment, whereas hot flashes and shaking from low estrogen levels, although uncomfortable, are more of an annoyance and can be corrected without entering the ICU.

Too much alcohol

In a study conducted in Spain, 3,285 people age 65 and older completed questionnaires on their drinking habits for three years. Those who drank an average of one or more alcoholic drinks a day had an increased risk of developing ET by 23 percent.[4]

Environmental toxins

In two studies, one conducted in New York City and one in Turkey, an association was found between increased blood levels of lead and ET. The Turkey study associated increased blood-level concentrations with a fourfold increased risk of developing ET.[5] The risk is also higher for those who have had prolonged and/or high-level exposure to pesticides, herbicides, and toxic metals.

Excitotoxins

Certain food products act as neurotoxins. Because these food products "excite" neurons to death, Dr. Russell Blaylock, a neurosurgeon, labeled them "excitotoxins." Frequent ingestion of excitotoxins can cause shaking. The most common and most dangerous excitotoxins are artificial sweeteners and monosodium glutamate (MSG).

Nutritional deficiency

The nervous system is dependent on certain vitamins, minerals, and other nutritional supplements to function properly. Being deficient in nerve-supporting nutrients (omega-3 fatty acids, B vitamins, and magnesium) can result in tremors and other symptoms. Fixing the deficiency usually reverses the symptoms.

Mild cognitive impairment (MCI) or dementia

In a large population-based study of almost 4,000 people (the Neurological Disorders of Central Spain, or NEDICES), ET was found to be associated with MCI and dementia. Those with ET onset after age 65 were found 57 percent more likely to have MCI than controls, whereas those with ET onset prior to age 65 were equally likely as the controls to develop MCI.[6]

Chronic stress and depression

The NEDICES study also linked chronic stress and depression to ET.[7] Whether someone is at higher risk of developing ET due to these conditions or whether ET encourages them needs further research.

Hearing impairment

In a study of 504 patients (250 patients with ET, 127 patients with PD, and 127 normal controls), the patients with ET were found to have increased hearing disability compared to the patients with PD and normal controls. Hearing loss in the ET group was also associated with tremor severity.[8]

Frailty

Core components of frailty from recent work by several groups included impaired grip strength, slowed gait, and low body-mass index (BMI). In the NEDICES study, those with ET were found to be frailer than their counterparts without the condition.[9] In another study, those with increased frailty were also more likely to develop dementia.[10]

3

Symptoms

TREMORS CAN RANGE from minor to severe. They may be so minor that they do not affect one's life, or they may be severe enough to interfere with normal activities. Common symptoms of ET may include one or more of the following:[1, 2, 3]

1. Difficulty writing, drawing, drinking from a cup, or using tools due to shaking. This symptom is the most common, since the arms and hands are the most frequently affected body parts.
2. Tremors when one is moving but less noticeable at rest. Shaking is not common when at rest, especially during sleep.
3. Uncontrollable head nodding. Motion is usually in a "yes-yes" or "no-no" movement. Head nodding does not happen to everyone but becomes more common as the disease progresses.
4. Shaking or quivering sound to the voice. In those where the tremors affect the voice box, a quivering sound to the voice becomes more common as the disease progresses.
5. Tremors come and go, but frequently get worse with age.
6. Tremors get better after drinking alcoholic beverages but may get worse after too much alcohol.

7. Tremors can be triggered or aggravated by certain medications, emotional stress, fatigue, hunger (low blood sugar), caffeine, cigarette smoking, or extremes of temperature.
8. Tremors usually begin on one side of the body and don't affect both sides in the same way.
9. Tremors in legs or feet and mild gait disturbances or balance problems. These are, however, rare. They may also be indicative of another medical condition.

4

Diagnosis

T O MAKE A diagnosis, a doctor should complete a physical exam and ask questions related to medical and personal history. The doctor should ask about a patient's history of smoking, drinking alcohol, prescription drugs, anxiety or nervous disorders, and sleep problems. There are usually no problems with coordination or mental function in those with ET. The diagnostic tests discussed below should also be performed. These steps are important to rule out reasons for shaking other than ET. A careful exam is critical to prevent a misdiagnosis. Some medications for Parkinson's disease are useless for ET.

Imaging studies
A CT scan of the head, brain MRI, and X-rays should be performed to detect tumors, evidence of stroke, and any other abnormalities that could cause tremors.

Blood tests
Blood tests should include a comprehensive metabolic panel (CMP), complete blood count (CBC), C-reactive protein (CRP), and thyroid panel.

Tests to measure blood levels of copper, magnesium, and vitamin B12 should also be included.

A CMP provides information about the current status of the metabolism, including the health of the kidneys and liver, as well as electrolyte and acid/base balance and levels of blood glucose and blood proteins. A CBC provides an overall picture of the blood, screening for a wide variety of conditions including anemia, bleeding disorders, infections, and leukemia. A fasting blood glucose is included with the CMP and is used to screen for pre-diabetes (insulin resistance) and diabetes.

A CRP test measures inflammation in the body. Anyone over the age of 40 or who has a chronic condition should take it.

A thyroid panel should include thyroid-stimulating hormone (TSH), free T4, and free T3. Many doctors will order TSH only. Free T3 is the most active form of thyroid hormone used by the cells in the body. However, the majority of thyroid hormones produced by the thyroid are T4, which need to be converted to T3. If your body isn't properly converting T4 to T3, TSH and T4 can indicate normal thyroid levels, while free T3 indicates low thyroid levels. Also, if your TSH test results indicate hyperthyroidism or hypothyroidism, free T4 can help define its severity. Hyperthyroidism, although not as common as hypothyroidism, can cause hand tremors.

Low levels of vitamin B12 or magnesium or high levels of copper can manifest in neurological problems.

A blood test for manganese should also be performed for those who've had manganese exposure, usually from working in the mining or welding industries.

Urine tests

Urine tests should include a urinalysis and a screening for heavy metals. A urinalysis aids in the detection of diabetes, kidney problems, infections, and many other conditions. Copper and lead should be part of the heavy metals screening test. Excessive levels of these metals could lead to tremors.

Wilson's disease

Wilson's disease is an inherited disorder that causes too much copper to accumulate in the brain, liver, and other organs. Symptoms are neuro-logical and psychiatric in nature. Normally, copper is absorbed from food, and any excess is excreted.

Blood and urine analyses are recommended to test copper levels. Brain scans, an eye exam, a biopsy of liver tissue, and genetic testing may also be desirable, depending on the level of signs and symptoms. Wilson's disease is fatal if left untreated, but if it is addressed, many peo-ple live normal lives with the disorder.[1]

Electromyography (EMG)

An EMG can help differentiate between PD and ET tremors by measuring the electrical activity within muscles. Listed below are the main differ-ences between the two conditions.

- In PD, shaking occurs when there is no movement or someone is at rest (tremors at rest), such as when the hands are on the lap or by the side. Shaking in ET usually happens *during* movement (action tremors), such as when writing or lifting a utensil. However, these conditions can overlap. Some studies show that 90 percent of Parkinson's patients have action tremors, and 20 percent of people with ET have tremors at rest.[2]
- The tremors in PD can affect the legs or feet, but they rarely do in ET.
- The legs of someone with PD become stiff and less flexible with time, but this does not occur in ET.
- The tremors rarely affect the voice and head in PD, but they can in ET.
- In PD, symptoms usually start on one side of the body and prog-ress to the other, whereas with ET, they usually affect both sides from the beginning. ET can start on one side of the body and

progress to the other side, usually within a couple of years, but this is less common.

- Drinking alcohol has no effect on the symptoms of PD but often improves the tremors in ET.
- Onset of ET is most common after age 65, whereas onset of familial ET is most common in early middle age. In PD, onset is most common between the ages of 55 and 65. However, both ET (including familial) and PD can start at earlier or later ages.

Part II

Conventional Treatments

5

Pharmaceutical Drugs

B ELOW IS A list of prescription drugs commonly used in the treatment of
ET. Approximately 60 percent of those with ET receive satisfactory
benefit from them. However, these medications cannot stop ET's progression and, like all drugs, come with their own set of problems and side
effects that are sometimes worse than the tremors themselves. Common
side effects of the following prescription drugs were obtained from www.
drugs.com (with permission). For a complete list of side effects for a particular drug, go to www.drugs.com and enter the drug's name.

Beta-blockers
Beta-blockers work by blocking nerve impulses to the muscles and are
commonly used to treat high blood pressure. Propranolol (Inderal) is
the only beta-blocker and medication approved by the Food and Drug
Administration (FDA) to treat limb and head ET.[1] Other beta-blockers that
may help with tremors are atenolol, metprolol, nadolol, and sotalol.

Common side effects of beta-blockers are usually mild, such as
fatigue and stuffy nose, but may include depression, erectile dysfunction,
slow heartbeat, and worsening of asthma. Although not common, propranolol can cause shaking, especially in children. Let your doctor know if

you have asthma, diabetes, heart problems, liver or kidney disease, or are pregnant before taking beta-blockers.

Anticonvulsants

Anticonvulsants, also known as antiseizure drugs, are used to treat seizures and sometimes anxiety and bipolar disorders. They work by increasing the inhibitory effects of GABA and thus suppress excitatory nerve-cell activity. Primidone (Mysoline) and topiramate (Topamax) are anticonvulsants commonly prescribed for the treatment of ET.[2]

Common side effects of Primidone include shakiness, trembling (ironically), unsteady walk, unsteadiness, or other problems with muscle control and coordination.

Topiramate (Topamax) has been shown to be effective in some, but many patients stop using it due to its adverse side effects that include dizziness, memory problems, nausea, numbness or tingling, trouble concentrating, and weight loss. To reduce the likelihood of side effects, most doctors recommend starting with a small dose at bedtime and gradually increasing from there.

Gabapentin (Neurontin) is a newer drug that has produced conflicting results in controlled studies.[3] It is prescribed for patients whose tremors are unmanageable with other medications. Common side effects include rolling eye movements and unsteadiness.

Perampanel (Fycompa) is currently in clinical trials to determine its effectiveness on tremors.[4] Common side effects include abnormal gait, aggressive behavior, ataxia, dizziness, drowsiness, equilibrium disturbance, falling, fatigue, headache, hostility, irritability, nausea, and sensation of spinning.

Antianxiety medications

These are used in patients who do not respond to other medications or have anxiety along with ET. These drugs are not as effective as beta-blockers and antiseizure medications, and they are addictive. Withdrawal symptoms are a risk if stopped suddenly. Commonly prescribed anti-anxiety drugs are alprazolam (Xanax), clonazepam (Klonopin), diazepam (Valium), and lorazepam (Ativan).

Common side effects of these drugs include confusion, dizziness, fatigue, feeling sad or empty, headaches, irritability, loss of coordination, memory problems, trouble concentrating, and trouble sleeping. In addition, a common side effect of clonazepam and diazepam is shaking and tremors (ironically).

Antidepressants
The antidepressant mirtazapine (Remeron) has been used for ET, but due to its lack of effectiveness and significant side effects, it is not frequently recommended. Common side effects include confusion, constipation, dizziness, drowsiness, dry mouth, frequent urination, headaches, increased appetite, nausea, and weight gain. Tremors are also a side effect of mirtazapine, but in less than 10 percent of patients.

6

Surgery

POTENTIAL CANDIDATES FOR surgical procedures are those for whom medications give unsatisfactory control of tremors and who have severe or disabling tremors that affect their ability to perform daily activities. We now have better understanding of brain anatomy, more detailed brain-imaging methods, and improved surgical techniques with fewer complications than when surgical treatments were first introduced.

Current surgical options for ET include deep brain stimulation (DBS) and thalamotomy. There are three types of thalamotomy surgical procedures, including stereotactic radiosurgery (SRS), radio-frequency thalamotomy (RF), and a new procedure called MRI-guided focused-ultrasound surgery (MRgFUS).

Deep brain stimulation

DBS is used to treat both ET and Parkinson's disease. It is FDA approved and has proven to significantly reduce tremors associated with ET. An electrical stimulator is used to quiet the overactive part of the brain, reducing tremor. Electrodes are implanted in the affected areas of the brain. The amount of stimulation is controlled by a pulse generator (a pacemaker-like device) placed under the skin near the clavicle. A wire under the skin connects this device to the electrodes in the brain. The device is programmed to deliver the proper amount of stimulation.[1]

Adverse side effects of DBS, as with any brain surgery, include cognitive changes (problems with confusion, mood, and speech), difficulty with walking or balance, hemorrhage, infection, paresthesia, stroke, and seizures.[2]

DBS requires more time and effort on the part of physicians and patients than RF thalamotomy. Permanent implantation of stimulating hardware (battery-powered neurostimulator, electrodes, and wire) requires frequent device reprogramming and battery replacement surgery about every three to five years. Hardware complications, such as wire breakage or dislocation and equipment failure, can also occur. In addition, the increasing use of wireless technology means that side effects from electromagnetic fields (EMFs) are becoming a serious consideration. Overstimulation and shock to patients with deep brain stimulators can happen if they are exposed to EMFs emitted from security systems, metal detectors, cell phones, smart meters, and other wireless devices. In spite of these issues, DBS, unlike RF, can be reversed if needed and has better outcomes than RF.[3]

Those who have significant memory problems or unstable medical conditions are not candidates for DBS; these conditions increase the risks associated with surgery. Those with health conditions that require repeated MRIs or full-body scans are also unlikely candidates.[4]

Stereotactic radiosurgery thalamotomy

SRS involves a specialized type of external therapy that pinpoints high doses of radiation directly onto a confined area with better accuracy than traditional radiation treatments. SRS is often referred to by the brand name Gamma Knife Radiosurgery. Gamma Knife has been used to target and destroy tumors, treat blood-vessel abnormalities, and destroy the brain cells that generate the hard-to-treat tremors of Parkinson's and ET. It is also used to treat trigeminal neuralgia, a painful facial condition. SRS takes approximately one hour, but the benefit may not be apparent until three to six weeks afterward.[5]

Gamma Knife offers a less invasive way to eliminate tremors than RF or DBS and is just as effective, according to the results of a long-term study that enrolled 183 patients with either Parkinsonian tremor or ET with hard-to-treat tremors. After a median of seven years subsequent to SRS treatment, researchers found that 83 percent of the Parkinson's patients and 87 percent of the ET patients had significant or complete reduction of tremors.[6]

Due to its lower risks, SRS is performed more than RF thalamotomy, but the procedure is usually restricted to patients with severe tremor who, because of unstable medical conditions, are not candidates for DBS.

Radio-frequency thalamotomy

RF is a procedure that destroys part of the thalamus to impede brain activity responsible for the tremors. It is performed under local anesthesia while the patient is awake. A small hole is drilled through the skull, and a thin wire electrode is inserted into the thalamus. A low-frequency current is then passed through the electrode to activate the tremors and confirm their location. The electrode is then heated to create a temporary lesion. The surgeon asks questions and performs tests to verify the location that is causing the tremors. The surgeon then creates a permanent lesion. Many patients experience complete relief or near-complete relief of symptoms.[7] But, unfortunately, RF has higher risk of serious side effects than SRS or DBS and so is used less frequently. Complications include bleeding, confusion, permanent balance or speech problems, cognitive impairment, and paralysis.[8]

MRI-guided focused-ultrasound surgery

MRgFUS is a new, noninvasive procedure that involves administering a series of focused ultrasound pulses through the patient's scalp and skull to a specific spot in the thalamus. The procedure can only be performed on one side of the body and takes about three hours. A pilot study of MRgFUS, led by W. Jeffrey Elias, MD, was performed on one patient at the University of Virginia (UVA). Positive results led to another clinical trial at UVA along with a study at the University of Toronto.[9]

From February to December of 2011, Dr. Elias performed phase one of the study at UVA. It involved 15 patients with severe ET. All showed improvements using MRgFUS. There were some minimal adverse side effects, including transient sensory, cerebellar, motor, and speech abnormalities in addition to persistent paresthesias (numbness and tingling) in four of the patients.[10]

Another study using MRgFUS was performed in Toronto, Canada, between May 2012 and January 2013 on four patients with chronic and medication-resistant ET. Their tremors were evaluated, and they received neuroimaging at the start of the study and at one month and three months after surgery. All showed immediate and sustained improvements, with an average symptom reduction in the treated hand of about 89 percent after one month and 81 percent at three months. They also had improved functional benefits, including in writing and motor tasks. One patient had postoperative paresthesia that persisted at the three-month evaluation, and another patient developed a deep-vein thrombosis (a blood clot in a deep vein) that was likely due to length of the procedure.[11]

MRgFUS was approved for treatment of ET by the FDA in July 2016. It was also approved in Canada, Europe, and Korea. However, the treatment is not covered by health insurance or medical payers in the United States or Europe.

—⟨⟩—

Before deciding on surgery, research the procedure you are considering and talk in detail with your surgeon. It is important to understand the benefits, expectations for the outcome, and the risks of any surgical procedure. Surgery is never to be taken lightly; get a second, third, or even fourth opinion. Don't agree to surgery until you feel comfortable with all aspects of it.

Bring a friend or family member to appointments. Meeting with surgeons is stressful. Someone else may think of questions to ask or remember information that you may have forgotten. Below is a sample list of questions.[12]

1. Am I a candidate for this procedure? Why or why not?
2. How does this procedure work?
3. How long does the procedure take? Does it require staying in the hospital?
4. What are the follow-up procedures after surgery?
5. Will the procedure cure or control my tremors, including head or voice tremors?
6. What are the risks of the surgery?
7. What is the risk of infection?
8. If the procedure will not cure my tremors, how much will it help?
9. Is there another option if this one doesn't work?
10. What are the potential benefits of this procedure?
11. What are the possible side effects of the procedure, and what percentage of people who get the procedure get each of the side effects?
12. What are my limitations after the procedure?
13. When can I go back to my normal activities, including work?
14. How many of these procedures have you done? What percentage was successful?
15. Can you connect me with other patients who have had the procedure?
16. If I have tremors in both hands, can a device be implanted on both sides at the same time for the DBS procedure, or does each one require a separate surgical procedure?
17. How long should the battery in the DBS procedure last? How is it replaced?
18. Will it be difficult to get through airport security when I fly? Will metal detectors (or Wi-Fi technology) interfere with the device?
19. Will there be limitations on having MRI or CT scans?

20. Will my insurance cover the procedure? Even if your doctor says that insurance will cover the procedure, always check with your insurance carrier to verify coverage, including for follow-up appointments. Get a quote in writing for total out-of-pocket costs for a worst-case scenario.

7

Other Options

BOTULINUM TOXIN (BOTOX), alcohol, and marijuana are other options for treating tremors. Botox is a powerful and potent poison that can paralyze the muscles and inhibit function of the parasympathetic nervous system, but it is significantly diluted for medical procedures, making it fairly safe. Botox is injected into the affected muscles and works by weakening muscle contractions, which helps reduce the severity of tremors. Botox has been most useful in the treatment of head, voice, and sometimes hand tremors.[1]

Side effects of botulinum toxin may include temporary paralysis of the injected muscle, flu-like symptoms, loss of appetite, and fatigue. Injections into the neck muscles for head tremors can cause temporary drooping of neck muscles. Sometimes the toxin can affect the swallowing muscles. In that case, patients need to mash or liquefy their food for a few weeks.[2] The downside of Botox injections is the expense, since insurance usually doesn't cover them. Injections need to be repeated every two to three months and can cost several hundred dollars each. Check with your insurance for coverage if you are considering this option.

Drinking alcoholic beverages responsibly—that is, having one or two drinks before social events—has been shown to reduce tremors for one to two hours. However, more severe tremors can recur after the effects of the alcohol have worn off.[3] After a while, using alcohol to reduce tremors can lead to excessive drinking, which can exacerbate tremors and defeat its purpose. Other side effects of alcohol consumption include addiction, balance problems, liver damage, and memory loss. This is why most doctors do not recommend drinking alcohol as a treatment for tremors.

Marijuana has also been shown to be helpful for those with anxiety and other central nervous system disorders in the short term. Like alcohol, however, marijuana has many side effects including addiction, depression, impaired mental abilities, mood disorders, and respiratory problems. As with alcohol, few doctors recommend marijuana for treating ET.[4]

Part III

Natural Remedies

Food Choices

NR1

Fear Frankenfoods

The center of the supermarket is for boxed, frozen, processed, made-to-sit-on-your-shelf-for-months food. You have to ask yourself, "If this food is designed to sit in a box for months and months, what is it doing inside my body?" Nothing good, that's for sure.

~Morgan Spurlock

"FRANKENFOODS" ARE FOODS that have been genetically engineered (GE) to produce specific characteristics such as increased yield, added nutrients, or resistance to herbicides. Foods that contain artificial growth hormones or that have been significantly changed through hybridization are also commonly referred to as frankenfoods.

Since the mid-1990s, when GE foods and artificial hormones were introduced into the food supply, many chronic conditions have increased significantly, including Alzheimer's (AD), autism, celiac disease, dementia, diabetes, inflammatory bowel disease (IBD), lupus, MS, obesity, PD, and certain cancers.[1, 2, 3, 4] Whether GE foods and artificial hormones are solely to blame remains to be proven. Electromagnetic fields have also increased significantly during the same period, mostly due to the increased use of cell phones and other electronics.

Due to a lack of studies, no link has yet been established between frankenfoods and symptoms of ET. However, ET is a nervous system disorder, and with neurological conditions on the rise, it is best to err on the side of safety and avoid frankenfoods.

Genetically Engineered (GE)

GE foods entered the food supply in 1996. Corn (except popcorn), soy, cottonseed oil, beet sugar, canola (rapeseed) oil, papaya, crookneck squash, and zucchini have all been genetically engineered.

About 90 percent of all corn, soy, cottonseed oil, and sugar beets grown in the United States has been genetically modified (GM) to resist glyphosate, a widely used herbicide. This way, more herbicides can be sprayed on crops to kill the weeds without harming the desirable plants. Your summer sweet corn has a very high chance of having been genetically modified and heavily sprayed with herbicide.

GM foods have never been properly tested for safety. Over 60 countries require labeling of GM foods including Australia, Brazil, China, Japan, Russia, and the 28 nations in the European Union, but not the United States. We are guinea pigs for multinational biotechnology corporations. Until GE foods in the United States are labeled (a girl can dream), the only way to avoid these crops is to buy those labeled USDA organic or from a trustworthy local farmer.

Canola oil has its own sordid history. There is no such thing as a canola plant. Canola oil is made from rapeseed and goes through a process of refining and bleaching that involves high temperatures and harsh chemicals. Traces of hexane (produced by refining crude oil) used in the refining process remain in the oil, even after considerable refining. Whether the oil is marked as organic makes no difference in the processing. Canola also contains erucic acid, which has been associated with fibrotic heart lesions. Although most of the erucic acid is removed during processing, some is left behind. It is best to play it safe and avoid canola oil entirely.

Papaya grown in Hawaii has been genetically modified to resist the ringspot virus. However, most papaya purchased within the continental United States comes from other countries whose papaya is not GE. Ironically for those who live in Hawaii, buying organic papaya is the only way to avoid the GE version.

About 15 percent of the crookneck and zucchini squashes on the market are genetically modified to resist viruses. Farmers have been resistant to plant these, so there's a good chance that what we buy is not GE. Without labeling, it is impossible to know for sure.

In November 2014, certain varieties of the russet potato were approved for genetic altering to reduce the amount of acrylamide produced when potatoes are fried. Acrylamide is a chemical suspected of causing cancer in people. Other more recent approvals by the FDA include GE apples (to prevent browning) in February 2015 and GE salmon (called AquaAdvantage) in November 2015.

AquaAdvantage salmon, the first GE animal, combines genes from a larger unrelated Pacific salmon and an Arctic eelpout to grow bigger and faster. GE salmon has not been properly tested on humans and will not be labeled, so the unsuspecting public will be taking unknown risks. Wild-caught salmon is not genetically modified, but most of it comes from the Pacific Ocean. Unfortunately, there is another problem with Pacific fish. Since the nuclear accident at Fukushima, Japan, in 2011, an estimated 300 tons of radioactive water has poured into the Pacific daily. The effect on wildlife is grave. Fish and mammals are washing up on the western shores of the United States and Canada. High levels of radioactive isotopes have been found in fish samples in the sea around Japan. If you consume fish, take a precautionary approach and avoid any food (fish, seaweed, miso, snack foods, and produce) coming from the Japan area and limit your intake of any other Pacific fish.

Another concern regarding GE foods is consuming meat, dairy, and eggs from animals that are fed GE corn or soy. There are no studies regarding the safety of consuming these products. It is wiser to eat less meat from organically raised animals than more from animals question-ably raised. Legumes, nuts, and seeds can be substituted for meat and dairy with no loss in nutrition. Protein is also found in most vegetables and whole grains.

Artificial Growth Hormones

Recombinant bovine growth hormone (rBGH) is a synthetic, man-made hormone that the FDA approved in 1993 for marketing to dairy farm-ers, mainly to increase milk production in cows. It is also referred to as recombinant bovine somatotropin (rBST) or artificial growth hormone. The European Union, Canada, and some other countries have never per-mitted the use of rBGH.[5] Milk from rBGH-treated cows has been found to have increased levels of the hormone insulin-like growth factor (IGF-1). Researchers have found that increased levels of IGF-1 significantly increase the risks of developing breast, colorectal, and prostate cancers.[6] In addition, girls are developing and going through puberty at earlier ages than they did 20 to 30 years ago. Could growth hormones in dairy and beef be the culprit?

Another concern is the increased use of antibiotics in cows treated with rBGH, who tend to develop more udder infections (mastitis) than untreated cows. Farm-raised chickens and fish are also treated with anti-biotics. Many researchers believe that these practices contribute to the current increases in antibiotic-resistant bacteria and superbugs.

Frankenwheat

The average American consumes over 125 pounds of wheat per year—equivalent to about 200 loaves of bread, or about half of a loaf per day. Both whole and white wheat are high-glycemic grains. High-glycemic foods increase blood glucose and inflammation in the body through advanced-glycation end products (AGEs). AGEs are substances that cause aging by stiffening arteries, clouding eye lenses, and killing neu-rons through oxidative stress. AGEs are implicated in many diseases and conditions, including Alzheimer's, cataracts, diabetes, cancer, dementia, and cardiovascular disease.

Gluten is a protein found in wheat, barley, rye, and oats. Oats do not naturally contain gluten, but they are usually processed in factories where wheat and other gluten-containing grains are processed. The gluten content of modern wheat grain is very high because it has been manipulated and hybridized over the past 50 years to increase gluten and shorten the grain for easier harvesting. The higher gluten content makes it more pliable, easier to handle, and tastier. No one can deny the irresistible draw of freshly-baked wheat bread. Originally, the wheat industry's goal was to sell more wheat and serve the millions of starving people around the world. However, this new dwarf wheat's higher gluten content is more difficult to digest for most (and impossible for some) than that of the wheat our ancestors consumed. Some have dubbed this new dwarf wheat "frankenwheat."

Gluten has been linked to Alzheimer's, autism, autoimmune disease, brain fog, cancer, dementia, depression, diabetes, fatigue, heart disease, migraines, mood swings, nerve damage, obesity, and PD. For two women who had been misdiagnosed with Alzheimer's disease, going on a gluten-free diet restored their memories.[7]

For those with the autoimmune condition called celiac disease, all gluten is impossible to digest, not just gluten from modern wheat. Unless diagnosed and treated, those with celiac disease can irreversibly damage their intestines and make it difficult for nutrients to be properly digested, putting them at high risk for malnutrition and other chronic diseases. Celiac disease cannot be reversed, but the damaging effects are reversible with complete abstinence from all gluten in the diet. An estimated 1 percent of people have celiac disease.

A less serious and more common condition related to grain consumption than celiac disease is gluten intolerance, also referred to as gluten sensitivity. It's not known how many people have this condition because its symptoms are largely unreported or are mistaken for those of other conditions.

Some people may also be allergic to wheat but not gluten itself, or they may have a problem with modern wheat but not other gluten-containing grains. These people must avoid modern wheat but can consume low-gluten grains like spelt, einkorn wheat, barley, and oats with no problem—myself included. Unlike wheat, spelt and einkorn have remained agriculturally unchanged.

No studies have targeted links between gluten or wheat and ET, but one has linked PD with gluten sensitivity. Having ET increases risk of developing PD, so an indirect link may exist between ET and gluten sensitivity. Some people with ET have reported reduction or elimination of tremors after going gluten free. At least three months may be needed to clear the effects of gluten from the body.[8]

Another good reason to eliminate gluten is its link to belly, or visceral, fat. Visceral fat is the fat that accumulates around the organs in the abdominal area. Gliadin proteins unique to wheat act as appetite stimulants, according to Dr. William Davis, author of the book *Wheat Belly*. Davis states that eating wheat provokes a fat-storing insulin response. Visceral fat triggers inflammation, which is the underlying factor for diabetes, hypertension, and heart disease in addition to dementia, rheumatoid arthritis, and colon cancer.[9] Cutting out wheat may also improve symptoms of acid reflux and irritable bowel syndrome (IBS) in some people.[10]

Visceral fat has also been linked to brain shrinkage and cognitive decline. According to one study of middle-aged men, the larger the belly, the smaller the volume of the brain and the higher the risk of dementia.[11] We all have enough problems without worrying about our brains shrinking.

The only way to give up gluten is to get anything containing it out of the house. Frankenwheat is very addicting. In a weak moment, a loaf of bread or box of cookies can disappear. I've experienced that magic act in my own home. Convince others who live with you to go along with the healthier, gluten-free diet. If not, tell them they need to get their wheat fix when away from home.

There are plenty of gluten-free foods, including fruits, vegetables, organic meats, nuts, tofu, and grains such as rice, quinoa, millet, and gluten-free oats. There are some good-tasting gluten-free processed products on the market, including those by the brand Amy's, but most are expensive and have a high glycemic index, so eat these sparingly.

Because frankenwheat is so addicting, withdrawal symptoms when one stops eating it are common. These can include bloating, constipation, depression, fatigue, headaches, and nausea. So give yourself a few weeks to a few of months to adjust to the new diet. After three months, you can add back some products made with low-gluten grains such as einkorn, barley, and spelt. Don't go overboard. If your symptoms return, it may indicate that you have a more severe gluten intolerance or even celiac disease. There are tests for gluten intolerance and celiac disease, but unfortunately, they are not always conclusive, and testing for celiac disease frequently involves an intestinal biopsy. However, if you feel great on a gluten-free diet, the tests are not necessary unless you want proof.

NR2

Eliminate Excitotoxins

Today, more than 95% of all chronic disease is caused by food choice, toxic food ingredients, nutritional deficiencies and lack of physical exercise.

~Mike Adams

THE NUMBER OF people getting neurodegenerative disorders is on the rise. Part of the reason has to do with the aging population. Other possible reasons include the explosion of EMF exposure (especially to Wi-Fi) in the past couple of decades and the use of excitotoxins in foods and drinks. (EMFs are discussed in detail in NR11.)

An excitotoxin is a substance that kills neurons by "exciting" them to death. The word "excitotoxin" was coined by Dr. Russell Blaylock, a neurosurgeon, in his book *Excitotoxins: The Taste That Kills*. Excitotoxins are dangerous because of their ability to cross the blood-brain barrier and destroy brain cells.

The destruction of neurons in different brain locations is evident in many modern-day diseases that include Alzheimer's, ALS, Huntington's, and PD. There is growing evidence that excitotoxins play a contributing role in these conditions and other disorders of the nervous system by accelerating the destruction of neurons. An injured or damaged brain is especially vulnerable. Excitotoxins can accumulate up to 72 hours after the incident.[1] This may explain the high incidence of NFL players with history of concussions who go on to develop Alzheimer's, chronic traumatic encephalopathy, or another neurodegenerative disease.[2]

Excitotoxins can cause or exasperate tremors. They are predominately found in artificial sweeteners and flavor enhancers.

Artificial Sweeteners

Probably the most toxic food ingredient (and most common artificial sweetener) on the planet is aspartame, the main ingredient of Equal and NutraSweet. Aspartame accounts for a significant amount of adverse reactions reported to the FDA for food additives. Some of these include aggression, anxiety, brain fog, confusion, depression, dizziness, insomnia, migraines, muscle spasms, nausea, restless-leg syndrome, seizures, severe *tremors*, slurred speech, and weight gain.[3]

The effects of aspartame can be inconspicuous and cumulative and develop over years or decades. Many diseases and conditions have been triggered or worsened by aspartame, including Alzheimer's, ALS, birth defects, cancer, chronic fatigue syndrome, diabetes, epilepsy, fibromyalgia, MS, and PD.[4]

Aspartame is found in most diet drinks and many low-calorie foods, including candy, cereals, cocoa mixes, chewing gum, gelatin mixes, instant flavored coffee mixes, instant tea beverages, laxatives, yogurts, and milk drinks. It is also found in some multivitamins and prescription drugs.

Since aspartame's approval by the FDA in 1981 for dry food and 1983 for soft drinks, obesity in America has significantly increased. Recent studies have shown that people who drink diet soft drinks have more difficulty losing weight than those who don't. The artificial sweetener tricks the metabolism into thinking it is getting real sugar which causes the body to release insulin and store it as belly fat. It doesn't matter that the sweetener is fake. The sweet taste still triggers a hunger response in the brain. There's no signal to tell you when to stop eating—so you don't. The result is weight gain (along with a few less brain cells), the opposite goal of most people who consume low-calorie products.

In one study, at the University of Iowa, diet soft drinks were found to increase risk of heart disease in older women. According to the study, led by Ankur Vyas, MD, researchers found that postmenopausal women who consumed two or more diet drinks a day were 30 percent more likely to experience a cardiovascular event and 50 percent more likely to die from related cardiovascular disease than women who never, or only rarely, consumed diet drinks.[5]

Let's dig a little deeper and see what makes aspartame so much more dangerous to health than what was previously mentioned. Aspartame breaks down in the body to three major components: methanol, aspartic acid, and phenylalanine. Aspartame is about 10 percent methanol by weight. Methanol (also known as methyl alcohol or wood alcohol) is a colorless, poisonous, and flammable liquid that can be inhaled from vapors, absorbed through the skin, and ingested. Methanol is a dangerous neurotoxin and known carcinogen and is the type of alcohol that can blind you if you drink it. Besides causing retinal damage in the eye, methanol interferes with DNA replication and causes birth defects.[6] Its breakdown components are formaldehyde and formic acid. Formaldehyde is highly toxic and a known carcinogen. Methyl alcohol is present naturally in higher amounts in fruits and vegetables, so why is it a problem in aspartame and not in produce? Because methyl alcohol binds to the pectin in fresh produce and eliminates in the stool, never being digested. It is, however, released in high amounts in spoiled produce, which most people will not eat (hopefully).

The second ingredient in aspartame is aspartic acid (about 40 percent of aspartame by weight), a nonessential amino acid that excites nerve cells. Amino acids keep us healthy when in a protein chain, but the amino acid in aspartame has been separated and used as an "isolate," meaning by itself. As an isolate or free-form amino acid, aspartic acid can easily cross the blood-brain barrier[7] and can act like an excitotoxin, killing neurons in its path.

The third ingredient in aspartame is phenylalanine, another amino acid used as an isolate.[8] Aspartame is about 50 percent phenylalanine by weight. Diet sodas and foods are especially harmful to children with phenylketonuria (PKU), who cannot break down phenylalanine in their bodies. Phenylalanine builds up, resulting in damage to the brain and central nervous system.[9]

Aspartame is not the only artificial sweetener. Acesulfame-K (Sunett and Sweet One), sucralose (Splenda), and saccharin (Sweet'n Low and Sweet Twin) are some others. All have reported side effects, including anxiety, anger, depression, diarrhea, difficulty breathing, headaches, mental confusion, mood swings, and nausea.

Another recently discovered risk of consuming artificial sweeteners is glucose intolerance. In a study, the three most commonly used artificial sweeteners (aspartame, saccharine, and sucralose) were given to mice in water in amounts equivalent to those permitted by the FDA. Those that drank the artificially sweetened water developed glucose intolerance as compared to mice that drank either plain or sugar water. Repeating the experiment with different types of mice and different doses of the artificial sweeteners produced the same conclusion: aspartame, saccharin, and sucralose were somehow inducing glucose intolerance.[10] Those with glucose intolerance are at risk of developing type 2 diabetes.

Let's review. Diet soft drinks kill brain neurons, make it difficult to lose weight, and increase risk of heart disease, type 2 diabetes, and cancer. There is nothing in diet soft drinks that benefits the body except water. The water in diet soft drinks could save your life if you were in the desert dying of thirst, but even that is debatable. Drinking diet sodas, especially with caffeine, on an empty stomach are more likely to cause gastrointestinal (nausea or stomach pain) or neurological problems (dizziness, headaches, shaking, or panic attacks) than when they are ingested with food, especially for sensitive individuals. Products with artificial sweeteners have negative nutritional value, meaning they do more harm to your body than good. Spending money on such a product is just plain foolish.

You might know Michael J. Fox from the recently aired hit show *The Good Wife*. Prior to that, he starred in *The Michael J. Fox Show* in which he played a family man with PD, a condition he's had for over 20 years. If you are old enough, you may also remember him from the hit show *Family Ties* in the 1980s and the hit movie *Back to the Future* (1985). During that period, Michael was also in several Diet Pepsi commercials. *Rolling Stone* magazine interviewed him in 1987, asking Michael if he drank the soda he was promoting. He said yes—in fact, he drank a couple of liters a day. Michael was diagnosed with PD at the young age of 30. Even if the aspartame in the Diet Pepsi was not the direct cause of Michael's PD, it may have triggered the disease at a much younger age than he would otherwise have developed it.

Some people who regularly drink diet soft drinks have reduced or stopped their tremors just by eliminating the soda. At the very least, artificial sweeteners can trigger or make tremors worse. Eliminating them from your diet is one of the best things you can do to improve your health.

Flavor Enhancers

Monosodium glutamate (MSG) and cysteine are flavor enhancers added to food to emphasize natural flavors. Both are excitotoxins. MSG is made from kombu, a type of seaweed, and has been used as a food additive for decades in Chinese food, canned vegetables, soups, sauces, processed meats, and diet foods.

The FDA has classified MSG as "generally recognized as safe" (GRAS), but it has received complaints of chest pain, facial pressure or tightness, headaches, heart palpitations, numbness, nausea, sweating, and weakness.[11] Other reported symptoms are burning sensation, difficulty breathing, loss of balance, panic attacks, and *tremors*. MSG has the potential to trigger or worsen neurological diseases such as Alzheimer's, ALS, MS, PD, and ET because of its ability to cross the blood-brain barrier. Yet, it is still on the market.

MSG is frequently disguised with names like "hydrolyzed vegetable protein" or "HVP," "yeast extract," and "autolyzed protein." These ingredients are found in many processed foods, including vegan products. The following is a list of food ingredients that are likely to contain MSG[12]:

- Monosodium glutamate
- Hydrolyzed vegetable protein
- Hydrolyzed protein
- Hydrolyzed plant protein
- Plant protein extract
- Sodium caseinate
- Calcium caseinate
- Yeast extract
- Textured protein
- Autolyzed yeast
- Hydrolyzed oat flour

Hydrolyzed protein is protein that has been broken down, or hydrolyzed, into its component amino acids. Like MSG, hydrolyzed protein is used to enhance flavor in a wide variety of processed food products such as soups, sauces, chili, stews, hot dogs, gravies, seasoned snack foods, dips, and dressings. It is often blended with other spices to make seasonings that are used in or on foods. The chemical breakdown of proteins may result in the formation of free glutamate that joins with free sodium to form MSG. When added this way, the FDA does not require food labels to list MSG as a separate ingredient.[13]

Cysteine (L-cysteine), another flavor enhancer, is a nonessential amino acid frequently used by food manufacturers for chicken stock. It is also used in flour and bakery products as a conditioning agent. In large quantities, cysteine acts as an excitotoxin. In laboratory tests, it showed the same pattern of neuron destruction as glutamate when injected in rats.[14]

Homocysteine, a metabolic derivative of cysteine, is also an excitotoxin. Elevated blood levels of homocysteine have been shown to be a major indicator of inflammation and cardiovascular disease. Several studies have found that all Alzheimer's patients examined had elevated levels of homocysteine.[15]

As noted earlier, many Chinese restaurants use MSG in their food. Before ordering, you can ask to have it omitted, but don't expect all MSG to be gone from the order. Chinese restaurants purchase products like sauces that may already come with MSG. It is less of a hassle, safer, and cheaper to learn to cook Chinese food at home.

NR3

Opt for Brain-Healthy Fats

Of all the things I've lost, I miss my mind the most.

~Mark Twain

FATS ARE ALSO known as lipids, which are simply storage units composed of fatty acids. Types of lipids include triglycerides, phospholipids, and sterols.

Triglycerides

Triglycerides are the most common fats found in the body and in the diet. They are classified by their degree of hydrogen "saturation" and length of their molecules, or chain length. There are three types of triglycerides: saturated, monounsaturated, and polyunsaturated. Each type differs greatly in how it is digested and utilized by the body.

Saturated fats

Fatty acids are "saturated" when all available carbon bonds are fully loaded with hydrogen atoms, forming straight chains. They remain stable at high temperatures and do not go rancid easily. They are typically solid or semisolid at room temperature. Saturated fats can be short-chain (4 to 6 carbon atoms), medium-chain (8 to 12 carbon atoms), or long-chain (14 to 18 carbon atoms) fatty acids. Short- and medium-chain fatty acids (also known as short- and medium-chain triglycerides or SCTs and MCTs, respectively) are directly absorbed by the body for energy and are not stored as fat. Long-chain fatty acids (also know as long-chain triglycerides or LCTs), found in most meats, are more difficult for the body to break down and are predominately stored as fat. Butterfat contains about 30 percent SCTs and MCTs and 70 percent LCTs. Beef fat contains almost all LCTs and coconut oil contains almost all MCTs. What this all means is that it is more difficult to lose weight (or easier to put weight on) consuming butter and beef fat than it is consuming coconut oil. In fact, coconut oil can actually aid in weight loss if it is substituted in the diet for animal fats and vegetable oils.

Saturated fats compose over 50 percent of cell membranes. They enhance the immune system and are essential for development of the brain in babies and children. Most people have been led to believe that consuming all fats, particularly saturated fats, will make them fat. This is why many popular diets are designed to eliminate saturated fats and significantly lower all others. This myth has been difficult to shake since the 1950s, when Ancel Keys proposed that cholesterol and saturated fats were mainly responsible for heart disease. Keys collected data from 22 countries but cherry-picked only 6 countries to support his theory. Had Keys included all 22 countries, the correlation between fat, cholesterol, and heart disease would have disappeared.[1]

Based on the purported "results" of Key's study, millions of people altered their diets by eating less meat, butter, eggs, coconut oil, and palm oil in the false hope of lowering their risk of heart disease. Worse yet, they replaced these items with margarine, vegetable oils, and more carbohydrates, mostly in the form of breads and other products that contain frankenwheat. All of these products have since been shown to contribute to heart disease.

Several current studies have found no link between saturated fats, cholesterol, and heart disease.[2, 3] In about 30 percent of the population, eating cholesterol-rich foods increases the concentration of high-density lipoprotein (HDL), or "good" cholesterol, in the blood. It has little or no effect in the rest of the population.[4] Yet people continue to consume vegetable oils and excessive carbohydrates because it is difficult to dispel myths that have been in place for decades.

The healthiest saturated fats are found in coconut and palm oils. Coconut and palm oils contain high levels of lauric acid, an MCT. As mentioned above, MCTs are rapidly absorbed by the body and quickly metabolized as fuel. MCTs supply the brain with energy and are essential for proper brain growth, which may explain why they are found in human breast milk. Lauric acid has been shown to be antibacterial, antiviral, and anti-inflammatory. Grass-fed butter and raw milk also contain lauric acid but in much smaller amounts.

The secret of MCTs is ketones, which the body makes directly from MCTs when it breaks down fat for energy. Health benefits associated with ketones include protection against brain cancer, brain damage, depression, diabetes, headaches, hypoglycemia, seizures, and neurodegenerative diseases such as Alzheimer's, Parkinson's, Huntington's, and ALS. Ketones also support thyroid function.[5]

Coconut oil, which contains the richest source of MCTs, blocks the toxic effects of many chemicals including, but not limited to, aflatoxin, toxins emitted by E. coli, ethanol, MSG, streptococci, and staphylococci.[6] Its antibacterial properties are the main reason why it is used in a procedure called oil pulling to help prevent and reverse gum disease (See Appendix B for more information). Coconut oil is also rich in polyphenols, substances that act as antioxidants.

Coconut oil remains stable when cooking at high temperatures, and it has a long shelf life of up to three years. Organic virgin coconut oil has much higher levels of MCTs than refined, hydrogenated, or powdered forms, which should all be avoided. Coconut oil can be used in cooking, baking, smoothies, soups, sauces, casseroles, and in hot cereals or taken by the spoonful as a supplement. When using it in baking, make sure that the other liquids in the recipe are at room temperature or warmer. Coconut oil solidifies at about 76 degrees or lower, so it will congeal when combining with cold ingredients.

Butter contains less lauric acid than coconut oil, but it has other benefits. It contains vitamins A, D, E, and K, and lecithin, an ingredient that helps lower cholesterol and support healthy brain cells. Like all healthy fats, butter calms the nervous system. It also supports adrenal and thyroid functions. The best butter is raw, organic butter made from the milk of grass-fed cows. Next is pasteurized butter from grass-fed cows, followed by regular pasteurized butter from cows raised without artificial hormones. All other butters have artificial hormones, unless labeled otherwise. Butter burns easily, so use it when cooking at low to medium temperatures. Coconut oil is preferred when cooking at medium to high temperatures. I try to use coconut oil for most of my cooking and baking, unless I want a buttery taste, like in cornbread.

What about palm oil? Nutritionally and environmentally, coconut oil is better. Palm oil is composed of 50 percent MCTs compared to 90 percent for coconut oil. It also has a strong and pungent taste. In addition, most palm oils are grown without use of environmentally sustainable measures. There are a few sustainable brands available, but they are very expensive.

Monounsaturated fats

Monounsaturated fats are missing a pair of hydrogen atoms, resulting in molecules that kink or bend at each double bond. They do not pack together as easily as saturated fats but are still relatively stable. Monounsaturated fats tend to be liquid at room temperature. Oleic acid, found in olive oil, is a monounsaturated fat. The oils in avocados, almonds, cashews, pecans, and peanuts also contain oleic acid.

Oleic acid, an omega-9 fatty acid, has been found in research to protect against heart disease, strengthen the immune system, reduce risk of cancer, and help manage blood-glucose levels. Consumption of olive oil, the pre-dominate oil used in the Mediterranean diet, has been associated with lower risk of rheumatoid arthritis and heart disease. A Mediterranean-style diet consists of high consumption of olive oil, legumes, whole grains, fruits, and vegetables; moderate consumption of fish and dairy products; and low con-sumption of meat. In one study, those who adhered to a Mediterranean-style diet had less risk of developing ET than those who did not.[7]

The diets of Italians, Greeks, and the French are high in fat-rich foods in the form of omega-3 and omega-9 fatty acids and saturated fats, yet their rate of heart disease and ET is lower than that of people in the United States. Furthermore, the French consume almost double the amount of saturated fats than do people in the United States, yet they have a much lower rate of death from heart disease. The French also consume signifi-cantly less polyunsaturated fats (and sugary food) in the form of marga-rine and soybean oil than we do in the United States.[8] More on these bad fats in the next section.

Monounsaturated fats have long-chain fatty acids that store as fat in the body if not needed for energy, so you might want to go easy on them if you are watching your weight. Extra-virgin olive oil has the best quality and taste. To get the most out of the nutrients in olive oil, use it in homemade salad dressings or on pasta instead of for frying. Olive oil oxidizes easily at high temperatures, so it is best to keep the temperature at medium or lower or use coconut oil instead.

Polyunsaturated fats

Polyunsaturated fats, also known as polyunsaturated fatty acids (PUFAs), are missing more than one pair of hydrogen atoms, resulting in molecules that don't pack together easily. They are found mostly in nuts, seeds, and fish. PUFAs remain liquid even when refrigerated. They go rancid easily, making them a poor choice for cooking, especially at medium to high temperatures. PUFAs contain omega-6 and omega-3 essential fatty acids (EFAs).

Omega-6 and omega-3 EFAs

EFAs are important for healthy blood vessels, nerves, and skin. They are abundant in brain tissue, providing the structural components of cell membranes in the brain, in addition to myelin, the fatty insulating sheath that surrounds each nerve fiber that enables it to carry electrical impulses or messages quickly and efficiently from cell to cell. If myelin is damaged, the impulses slow down, and a demyelinating disease can occur, such as MS. The sheath plays a critical role in ensuring proper function of the nervous system.

Alpha-linolenic acid (ALA) is the shorter-chain form of omega-3. It is the only omega-3 found in plants. Foods rich in ALA include rapeseeds (canola), flaxseeds, and walnuts. Longer-chain forms of omega-3, found mostly in animals, are eicosapentaenoic acid (EPA) and docosahexaenoic acid (DHA). There are high amounts of EPA and DHA in fish and shellfish. DHA is the primary structural component of the brain and the retina of the eye. DHA deficiency has been linked to ADHD, depression, and Alzheimer's disease, which is understandable, as DHA is so critical to neurological brain function.

Linoleic acid (LA) is the shorter-chain form of omega-6. It is the most prevalent PUFA in the Western diet, found in canola, corn, soybean, and sunflower oils. The longer-chain form of omega-6 is arachidonic acid (AA), which is an important constituent of cell membranes and a material the body uses to make substances that combat infection, regulate inflammation, promote blood clotting, and allow cells to communicate. AA is found in liver, egg yolks, animal meats, and seafood.

Omega-6 and omega-3 EFAs are both important to health, but must be balanced properly in the body. Prior to the popularity of processed foods that use vegetable oils and hydrogenated fats, Western diets contained a healthy ratio of omega-6 to omega-3 fatty acids of 1:1 to 2:1. The ratio today is closer to 20:1. This imbalance stimulates the body's production of inflammation-causing chemicals and free radicals. Studies show that excessive amounts of omega-6 polyunsaturated fatty acids (PUFA) and a very high omega-6/omega-3 ratio promote cancer, cardiovascular disease, and autoimmune and inflammatory diseases, whereas increased levels of omega-3 PUFA (a low omega-6/omega-3 ratio) reduce risk of developing these conditions. More specifically, a ratio of 2.5:1 reduced cell growth in patients with colorectal cancer while a ratio of 4:1 with the same amount of omega-3 PUFA had no effect. In addition, a ratio of 5:1 had a favorable effect on patients with asthma compared to a ratio of 10:1, which had adverse consequences. Lastly, a low ratio of omega-6/omega-3 curbed inflammation in patients with rheumatoid arthritis and was associated with reduced risk of breast cancer in women.[9]

Why are vegetable oils so bad for your health? Unlike olive or coconut oils, which can be extracted by cold pressing, vegetable oils are chemically extracted using chemical solvents. To make matters worse, some of these oils are subjected to yet another chemical process called partial hydrogenation. Partial hydrogenation is a process by which liquid vegetable oil is packed with hydrogen atoms and converted into a solid fat, giving it a long shelf life, high melting point, and a creamy texture. It has been the fat of choice for the food industry since the 1960s due to its low cost and long shelf life. Margarine, shortening, and most processed foods that contain fat are made with hydrogenated fats. What's more, if the products contain corn or soybean oils, they have the added bonus of containing GMOs (unless certified organic or non-gmo project verified).

Omega-3 EFAs have been shown to reduce anxiety and depression, two conditions that can trigger tremors. In a study conducted in 2008 using substance abusers, patients were given a high dose of EPA (greater than two grams per day). The results were a significant reduction in anxiety compared to those receiving a placebo. More importantly, the degree of anxiety reduced was highly correlated to the decrease of the ratio of omega-6 fats to omega-3 fats in the blood.[10] In other studies with normal individuals without clinical depression or anxiety, increased intake of omega-3 fats improved their ability to handle stress in addition to improving their mood.[11]

EPA is the primary anti-inflammatory omega-3 fatty acid for the brain. If levels of EPA are low in the blood, they are also low in the brain. To further complicate the matter, the lifetime of EPA in the brain is very limited.[12] Therefore, a constant supply of EPA is needed in the bloodstream to prevent inflammatory responses in the brain, which cause the formation of free radicals, eventually resulting in the death of brain neurons. It's not enough to eat more omega-3 EFAs; the amount of omega-6 EFAs in the diet must also be reduced. Animal studies show that if the brain is fed loads of fish oil followed by a pile of bad fats, protection from dementia is reduced.

To keep brain neurons healthy and to reduce stress levels, inflammation, and tremors, a ratio of omega-6 to omega-3 EFAs should range from 1:1 to 3:1. To reduce omega-6 consumption, get rid of all junk foods, margarines, vegetable oils, shortenings, and anything with trans-fatty acids, or hydrogenated fats. Hydrogenated fats are found in many processed foods, including nondairy creamers, salad dressings, cakes, cookies, and breads, so read ingredient labels closely.

After cleaning your house of the bad fats, purchase foods that contain high levels of omega-3 EFAs such as wild-caught salmon, white fish, eggs, flaxseeds (or flaxseed oil), pumpkin seeds, and walnuts. As mentioned earlier, due to unknowns about the Fukushima nuclear disaster, fish consumed from the Pacific should be limited. Fish caught wild from the Atlantic are safer to eat, but all fish have varying levels of pollutants. Smaller fish like salmon and cod have the lowest levels of pollutants. Farm-raised fish should also be avoided. Fish farms use hormones to help fish grow faster and pesticides to keep the water clean from high levels of pollutants including fish feces. Like factory-farmed animals, fish in close quarters get stressed and sick more often, so some farmers use antibiotics to prevent illness. In addition, they are frequently fed GMO grains (corn and soy) with colorants added (artificial dyes) to make them appear more appetizing. Grain-fed fish also have lower levels of omega-3 EFAs and higher levels of omega-6 EFAs than wild-caught fish.

A squirrel's first choice for food is nuts and seeds and for a reason. They are packed with nutrients. Walnuts have the highest levels of omega-3s, but almonds, cashews, and Brazil nuts have higher levels of calcium and magnesium, making them great for preventing osteoporosis and relaxing the nervous system. Besides omega-3 EFAs, pumpkin seeds are high in magnesium and zinc. Nuts and seeds are also high in antioxidants, protein, and fiber. For optimum nutritional benefits from these little power houses, eat a variety (about a handful) of nuts and seeds every day. Store them in the refrigerator to prevent their oils from going rancid.

Omega-3 EFAs can also be taken as a supplement in the form of fish oil, flaxseed oil, marine microalgae, or krill oil. Make sure that any fish or cod liver oil is purified to eliminate environmental pollutants such as PCBs, which are man-made chemicals persisting in the environment after heavy use in industry from 1929 to the 1980s. They can collect in the body damaging the thyroid and many other organs. PCBs can also cause cancer due to their high chlorine content.

Flaxseed oil is the preferred option of omega-3 fatty acids for vegans and vegetarians. Flaxseed does not contain either DHA or EPA like fish oil. Instead, it contains ALA, which must be converted to EPA in the body to be useful. This means that higher amounts of flaxseed (at least twice as much) are needed because the body does not convert all ALA to EPA. According to one study, one group of participants received 1.2, 2.4, or 3.6 grams of flaxseed oil while another group received 1.2 grams of fish oil. Their blood was tested every 2 weeks for 12 weeks. It took at least 2.4 grams of flaxseed oil for blood levels of EPA to rise in that group, but both EPA and DHA rose in the group that took 1.2 grams of fish oil. In addition, the ALA did not appear to convert to DHA in the body at all.[13]

Marine microalgae might be the best vegetarian source of omega-3 fatty acids; they are packed with antioxidants and other nutrients. Spirulina and chlorella blue-green algae are examples of dietary supplements that have been used to promote healthy brain function, detoxification, and immune-system support. Marine microalgae come in softgels, capsules, tablets, powders, and liquids.

Lately, there has been a lot of buzz about the benefits of krill oil as an omega-3 supplement. Unfortunately, the only research on its benefits was done by a company that also sells the product. Furthermore, according to National Geographic, the supply of krill is shrinking in the Antarctic due to overfishing. Krill are tiny, shrimplike crustaceans that hundreds of animals, including whales, rely on as their main source of food. There is no need to take an unproven supplement or endanger wildlife when there are other food options of omega-3 fatty acids available.

See Appendix E for dosage and brand recommendations for omega-3 EFA supplements.

Phospholipids

Phospholipids are a class of lipids that form the plasma of cells. Unlike triglycerides, which are formed with three fatty acid groups attached to a glycerol molecule, phospholipids are formed with two fatty acid groups and a phosphate group attached to a glycerol molecule. Phosphatidylcholine (PC), phosphatidylinositol (PI), and phosphatidyl-serine (PS) are the most common phospholipids. Choline (part of PC) and inositol (part of PI) are both considered B vitamins. Serine (part of PS) is an amino acid.

Phospholipids help brain cells communicate. Like omega-3 EFAs, they are important for optimal brain health and cognitive function. The body makes acetylcholine from PC or choline. PS strengthens cell membranes, which helps improve attention span, memory, and mood. It can also help raise acetylcholine levels. Acetylcholine is a neurotransmitter that is important for learning and memory. Significant deficiencies are associated with Alzheimer's and dementia. Adequate amounts of phospholipids can be easily obtained through diet. Food sources of these nutrients are eggs, liver, soy, peanuts, and wheat germ. Smaller amounts can be found in grains, vegetables, and fruits. PC and PS supplements have been used in treating ADHD, memory problems, and depression. Choline-containing phospholipids are important in the treatment of ET. There is more discussion on this topic in NR17.

Sterols

Sterols are unsaturated solid alcohols having the structure of a steroid. They are found in the tissues of animals, plants, and fungi. Cholesterol, the most abundant sterol, is found in animals. Phytosterol is a cholesterol-like steroid found in plants, and ergosterol is a sterol found in fungi. Ergosterol is used to make vitamin D2, a vegan form of vitamin D.

Cholesterol

Cholesterol is a soft, waxy substance found in the bloodstream and every cell in the body. Cholesterol maintains the integrity of cell membranes, synthesizes bile acids for digestion, and helps to make vitamin D and steroid hormones like cortisol, estrogen, and testosterone.

Some of the cholesterol in the body is made by the liver, and some is obtained through diet. High-density lipoprotein (HDL) is considered the "good" cholesterol and low-density lipoprotein (LDL) the "bad" (although this is somewhat of an oversimplification). The main function of LDL is to transport cholesterol from the liver to the cells of organs and tissues. HDL carries cholesterol that had been discarded by the body's cells back to the liver for recycling or excretion. Recycled cholesterol can break down fat consumed or help to produce hormones. The brain and nervous system also use it to form synapses, the connections between neurons. Even though the brain is only 2 percent of total body weight, it contains 25 percent of the body's cholesterol. Therefore, learning, thoughts, imagination, and memories are dependent on cholesterol.

Both LDL and HDL are essential for good health. LDL particles are safe and healthy when they are large and buoyant. They are only dangerous when they are small and dense. The small particles can pass through the cells of the arterial lining and accumulate on arterial walls, leading to thick, hard arteries, a condition referred to as atherosclerosis. People who have small, dense LDL particles have three times the risk of heart disease.[14] The main cause of small, dense LDL particles is oxidation, which occurs as a result of inflammation, chronic stress, high blood sugar, poor nutrition, toxins, and lack of physical activity. The LDL particle test (also referred to as NMR lipid profile, or NMR lipoprofile) measures the number, size, and density of LDL particles. High LDL levels are the body's way of maintaining the correct balance. Damaged LDL is turned into plaque, which the blood platelets use to produce the cholesterol sulfate that the heart and brain need for optimal function. What this also means is that when cholesterol is lowered artificially with a statin drug, plaque may effectively be reduced, but this doesn't address the root problem and results in deficiency of cholesterol sulfate and increased risk of a heart attack.

In one study, progression of coronary artery calcification increased with statin use.[15] In another six-year study of over 47,000 patients treated with a statin drug, the lowest mortality rates were seen in patients with total cholesterol levels between 200–259 mg/dl. Those with total cholesterol levels between 200–219 mg/dl had a lower rate of heart disease than those with higher or lower levels. People with total cholesterol levels below 160 had the highest death rates.[16] Another study, in Sweden, that followed 289 municipalities from 1998 to 2002 found no correlation between the increased use of statin drugs and incidence of acute myocardial infarction (AMI). Even though statin use increased significantly during that period, mortality from AMI remained constant.[17]

More about statin drugs

Most doctors believe that statin drugs have few side effects because few were reported in clinical trials. Statins were proven to be safe, well tolerated, and effective. How? Drug companies do just about anything to get their products successfully through clinical trials and to market. Trial participants are carefully screened to find basically healthy people with mild forms of the condition being studied, whereas those with serious problems, such as arthritis, cancer, dementia, diabetes, and heart, kidney, or liver disease are frequently excluded. Women of childbearing age are also excluded from trials. In addition, clinical trials have become shorter to get drugs on the market as soon as possible to "help" people.

Death from heart disease has decreased since the introduction of statin drugs in 1987, but this is more likely due to advances in detection, improvements in long-term and emergency care, life-saving surgeries, a decrease in smoking, and a decrease in infectious diseases rather than to statins.

Some of the side effects of statin drugs include birth defects, coenzyme Q10 (CoQ10) and hormone depletion, cataracts, difficulty sleeping, drowsiness, headaches, extreme fatigue, gastrointestinal problems, memory loss, muscle pain and damage, nausea and vomiting, total global amnesia (TGA), and erectile dysfunction (as if the other side effects weren't enough). A rarer side effect of taking statins is developing rhabdomyolysis, a disease causing severe muscle damage, kidney failure, and death.

Baycol, manufactured by Bayer AG, was one of the most dangerous cholesterol-lowering drugs on the market before Bayer voluntarily recalled it in 2001. Risk of developing rhabdomyolysis from Baycol was considered much greater by the FDA than taking other statins. Over 100 deaths and thousands of injuries have been linked to Baycol.

CoQ10 is a critical component of mitochondria, a type of organelle (a specialized cell part) responsible for producing the energy that cells need to do their job. CoQ10 is a potent antioxidant and required for a healthy heart. Since statin drugs hit the market, congestive heart failure has been rising. Depletion of CoQ10 by statins may be the reason.

Giving someone with dementia a statin drug is like injecting a diabetic with high-fructose corn syrup. TGA is a transient form of memory loss that can last from 15 minutes to half a day. Imagine this happening when you're flying an airplane, as the pilot and doctor, Duane Graveline, could have been doing when he got TGA. He wrote about his experience in *Lipitor: Thief of Memory*.

Babies need high amounts of cholesterol to develop normally. Birth defects from statins are not common, because only 3 percent of women of childbearing age take statins. However, in one study, 20 of 52 babies exposed to statins in the womb were born with birth defects.[18]

To be fair, there are some benefits to statin drugs. They have anti-inflammatory and anticlotting effects. Since inflammation is associated with heart disease, statin drugs can lower the risk, at least initially. And, of course, reducing blood clots can reduce risk of strokes. But are these benefits enough to outweigh the side effects? No, because there are safer ways to reduce inflammation without the use of statins. See Appendix D for details.

NR4

Steer Clear of Harmful Protein

Life expectancy would grow by leaps and bounds if green vegetables smelled as good as bacon.

~Doug Larson

HARMANE, A NEUROTOXIN found in animal protein that is produced when meat is cooked, has been shown to be one of the most potent tremor-producing beta-carboline alkaloids in lab tests with mice.[1] In a follow-up study, blood levels of harmane were found, on average, to be 50 percent higher in those with ET compared to controls.[2] In another study of 200 people, 100 with ET and 100 without, blood concentrations of harmane were elevated in cases of those with and without a family history of ET.[3]

Harmane levels are higher in meats that have been cooked at high temperatures for longer times, such as in barbecuing. Studies have not proven that those with ET eat more of these products. There may be something genetic about ET that predisposes them to collect higher levels of harmane in their blood. Further research is needed.

Not only does overcooking meat produce tremors, it increases risk of cancer due to increased free-radical formation. To be on the safe side, you should stay away from microwaving and barbecuing cooking methods, because they produce the highest amounts of harmane. Safer cooking methods include oven cooking and pan frying until medium rare instead of well-done and crispy.[4]

People eat meat mainly for its high levels of protein and the taste. Proteins are the primary building blocks of muscles, tendons, ligaments, organs, and glands. Every living cell and all bodily fluids (except bile and urine) contain protein. A certain amount of protein from the diet is mandatory for growth and development.

Amino acids are the building blocks of protein. The human body needs about 22 amino acids that are classified as either essential or nonessential. Essential amino acids cannot be manufactured by the body and therefore need to be obtained from diet. Nonessential amino acids are manufactured by the body. Animal products such as beef, pork, poultry, fish, eggs, and dairy contain complete proteins, meaning they contain all essential amino acids. Incomplete proteins contain some amino acids but not all. Foods with incomplete proteins include fruits, vegetables, legumes, and whole grains.

Most Americans get plenty of protein in the form of fast-food burgers, fried chicken, processed meats and cheeses, pasteurized milk, and ice cream. Unfortunately, most such products come from animals raised on factory farms, or concentrated animal-feeding operations (CAFOs). These animals live in horrific conditions and are given plenty of antibiotics and/or artificial growth hormones.

Consuming too many antibiotics in food can lower resistance to infections and may explain the increase in antibiotic-resistant bacteria and superbugs. Consuming artificial hormones found in today's beef and dairy increases risk of cancer and reproductive problems. The increase in artificial hormones may also explain the increasing rates of early puberty in children. The United States is one of few developed countries that allows milk and meat meant for human consumption to be treated with artificial growth hormones. They are banned in Australia, Canada, Japan, New Zealand, and the European Union.

Studies have shown that those who eat red meat have a higher risk of heart disease and cancer. It's no wonder when most cattle live in CAFOs, consume heavily pesticide-sprayed GE grains, and are injected with antibiotics and hormones. The poor diet and high stress from the animals' unnatural lifestyle weakens them and makes them sick. Cattle's digestive systems are meant for grazing on grass. When they eat grains (and sometimes meat by-products from other animals), many problems develop. One major problem is mad-cow disease, or bovine spongiform encephalopathy (BSE), a fatal neurodegenerative disease that has been transmitted to humans as Creutzfeldt-Jakob disease (CJD). The worse outbreak of CJD was in the United Kingdom in the mid-1980s. Approximately 80 people died from the fatal condition, over 179,000 cows had mad-cow disease, and another 4.4 million had to be killed as a precaution.[5]

CJD can take months to several years to show up, so the burger you eat today may kill you in two to eight years. Who is your family going to sue for your death then? There hasn't been a case of mad-cow disease in the United States for several years, but that doesn't mean consumers should entrust their health to large agricultural businesses. Factory-farmed cattle also have higher risk of developing E. coli and tumors than grass-fed cattle because of their diet. The saying "you are what you eat, eats" is so true.

Pastured cattle eat grass as they are meant to, live outdoors, and live longer lives because they are not shot up with growth hormones or live in stressed, crowded quarters. Grass-fed cattle are at much lower risk than factory-farmed cattle of developing disease. They also have a higher omega-3 to omega-6 ratio than factory-farmed cattle. Beef from organically raised, grass-fed cattle is much more expensive than beef from factory-farmed cattle; but it is better to eat grass-fed beef occasionally or not at all than to eat toxic meat from stressed and sick cattle.

Factory-farmed chickens are not any better off than factory-farmed cattle. Each chicken has a space about the size of copier paper to move around in. Due to the stress of these overcrowded conditions, the chickens peck and fight with each other, which has lead to the practice of debeaking chicks. Broiler chickens live for only a few months before hitting the slaughterhouse. Free-range chickens, if raised properly, live several years. But beware of the "free range" label. It can mean that the chickens see daylight for as little as one hour a day. Chickens raised organically (fed organic, non-GMO feed) have a better chance of being treated humanely because the farmer must spend money on certification and better-quality feed to obtain the "USDA Organic" label. The best option is to buy from a local farm where you can observe how the chickens are raised.

Pigs, one of the smartest animals alive, are treated just as poorly. They live in quarters so small that they are unable to turn around. Their meat is garbage because they will eat just about anything, including maggots. Pigs can also carry parasites and viruses. Organic, pasture-raised pork is available but is much more expensive.

Processed meats, such as luncheon meats, hot dogs, and bacon, contain nitrites, a substance known to cause cancer. Nitrate-free, organically-processed meats are costly and never as healthy as nonprocessed meats, so they should be eaten sparingly.

Abstaining from animal protein several days a week is good for the environment and your body. The methane and waste products from factory-farmed animals is a major contributor to air and water pollution. Eating animal meat is not necessary to obtain adequate amounts of protein in the diet; legumes, nuts, seeds, and whole grains are excellent sources.

—⟋⟍—

Note on microwave cooking

Are microwave ovens safe for cooking foods other than meat? There is much controversy regarding the use of microwave ovens. Those against microwaves say they change the molecular structure of food, rendering the nutrients inert and possibly carcinogenic.[6] But according to Harvard Health Publications, microwaves may actually keep more vitamins and minerals in the food because they heat food quickly and with less water than conventional cooking.[7]

Some opponents of microwaves point out the poor health of people who regularly use them. This probably has to do with the consumption of processed food products made specifically for microwaves than the device itself. So what can you do? I prefer to err on the side of caution and cook most of my meals on the stove top and only use a microwave for occasional reheating. If you consume nothing but microwaved foods, you should learn to cook healthier and tastier meals by taking a cooking class at your local culinary school or community college. It's fun and you get to eat what you create.

NR5

Choose Carbs Carefully

Very simply, we subsidize high-fructose corn syrup in this country, but not carrots. While the surgeon general is raising alarms over the epidemic of obesity, the president is signing farm bills designed to keep the river of cheap corn flowing, guaranteeing that the cheapest calories in the supermarket will continue to be the unhealthiest.

~MICHAEL POLLAN

CARBOHYDRATES (CARBS) ARE predominately found in plants or derived from plants. The body uses carbs to make glucose. The body can use glucose as fuel immediately or store it in the liver or muscles to use at a later time. Since the liver and muscles have limited storage room, continued intake of carbohydrates converts to fat in the body. Avoiding that process is the logic behind today's popular low-carb diets.

Carbs are commonly classified as either complex or simple. Complex carbs are made up of sugar molecules that are strung together in long, complex chains. They are found in foods such as legumes, whole grains, and vegetables. Complex carbohydrate foods provide vitamins, minerals, and fiber.

Simple carbs, on the other hand, have one or two sugars or short chains that break down very quickly in the body. Eating too many of these is a problem, because simple carbs are much more likely to turn to fat if the body cannot use them for energy quickly enough. Simple carbs include those found in fruit (fructose), milk (lactose), and refined products such as beet and cane sugar, corn syrup, white flours, white rice, and anything made with these ingredients. Refined carbs and products made from them are referred to as "empty" calories because they have little to no nutritional value. In fact, many are negative in nutritional value because of the damage they can create in the body.

Sweeteners such as sugar and high-fructose corn syrup (HFCS) are triggers for tremors because they stimulate the central nervous system and can cause low blood sugar, or hypoglycemia. Common symptoms of hypoglycemia are anxiety, confusion, dizziness, drowsiness, headaches, hunger, fatigue, general weakness, racing heart, *shaking or trembling*, sweating, vision changes, and an urgency to eat. Someone who has hypoglycemia usually cannot go more than a couple of hours without eating. Chronic hypoglycemia can lead to insulin resistance, a prediabetic condition, or diabetes.

Low-carb and low-glycemic diets can reverse and prevent hypoglycemia. A recent study comparing a low-carb to a low-fat diet found that the first is more effective for both losing weight and reducing cardiovascular risk.[1] Opinions vary on the numbers, but a healthy person can safely consume about 150 to 200 grams of carbs per day, depending on size. Those who are insulin resistant or diabetic should try to stay below 150 grams of carbs.

Glycemic index (GI) is a measure of how quickly glucose levels rise after eating a particular food. High-GI foods cause glucose and insulin levels to rise and are associated with type 2 diabetes and heart disease. Foods with a GI of 70, 56 to 69, and 55 or less are considered high, medium, and low, respectively. High-GI foods are often refined, such as white bread, white rice, cornflakes, bagels, pretzels, and HFCS. White potatoes are also a high-GI food. Foods with a medium GI are whole wheat, dried fruit, bananas, and table sugar. Foods with a low GI are brown-rice syrup, raw honey, beans, legumes, seeds, vegetables, certain whole grains, and some fruits. You can find many glycemic-index food-list charts on the Internet.

Because they break down at a much slower rate and don't convert to fat as readily, complex carbs are preferable to simple carbs. Complex carbs naturally contain vitamins, minerals, and antioxidants. Examples are legumes (beans, lentils, and peas), starchy vegetables (potatoes), nuts, seeds, and whole grains (brown rice, buckwheat, millet, oatmeal, and quinoa).

Brown rice is a good source of B vitamins, magnesium, phosphorus, and selenium. Unfortunately, researchers have discovered that it can also contain high levels of arsenic. Rice grown in Arkansas, Louisiana, Mississippi, Missouri, and Texas had the highest levels. Brown and white basmati rice grown by Lundberg in California had about 40 percent less arsenic on average than rice grown in other areas of the United States. Brown rice had more arsenic than white rice. White basmati rice from India and Jasmine rice grown in Thailand also had some of the lowest levels of arsenic.[2]

Brown rice has many more nutrients and a lower GI than white rice, so don't give up on it. To reduce exposure to arsenic, limit servings of brown rice to two (one serving is one cup) per week. Rinsing the rice thoroughly before cooking and boiling it in more water than is needed can reduce arsenic levels by approximately 30 to 40 percent according to research. Products made from brown rice—cookies, crackers, bread, flour, pasta, and ready-to-eat cereals—should be avoided or severely limited because they have some of the highest levels of arsenic. If you prefer white rice, limit servings to two per week and make sure it is eaten with protein to lower the GI.

A healthy diet should consist mostly of complex carbs, plus a small amount of nutrient-rich simple carbs from fruit. To prevent low blood sugar (hypoglycemia), eat carbohydrates, especially those with a low GI, with protein. For example, have a banana with peanut butter or a slice of whole grain toast with an egg.

HFCS is made with GM corn. It is especially dangerous because it blocks leptin, the hormone that signals satisfaction from eating. Without this signal, you never feel satisfied, so you keep eating. It is almost impossible to maintain a healthy weight while consuming moderate-to-high amounts of HFCS. In one study, lab rats, with access to HFCS, gained significantly more body weight over the course of several months than control groups. The weight gain was accompanied by an increase in abdominal fat and elevated triglyceride levels, thus suggesting that excessive consumption of HFCS may contribute to the incidence of obesity in humans.[3] HFCS is found in abundance in processed foods, fruit-flavored drinks, and soft drinks.

Diet soft drinks (as discussed in NR2) are not a better alternative. In a study in Texas of 474 participants, those who drank two or more diet sodas a day had waist sizes 500 percent greater than those who did not drink them at all.[4] Diet soft drinks have also been associated with an increased risk of type 2 diabetes.[5] In addition, many soft drinks contain artificial dyes, caffeine, and phosphoric acid. Caffeine can worsen tremors, and phosphoric acid is associated with lower bone density in women. Aspartame, HFCS, artificial dyes, caffeine, and phosphoric acid are five good reasons to avoid soft drinks.

Fruit drinks are not much better than soda. They are frequently made from HFCS or artificial sweeteners (if low calorie), artificial flavors, and other additives. Water is the best drink for the body. To make water more palatable, flavor it with a small amount of 100 percent fruit juice in a ratio of no more than one part juice to three parts water. The healthiest choices are those made from organic berries, pineapples, and/or pomegranates with no added sweeteners or artificial ingredients. If you want a sweetener, you can add little honey or stevia. Limit consumption of commercial apple and orange juices. Many apple juices are too concentrated in sugar and contain high levels of arsenic.[6] Commercially-sold orange juices, no matter what the label states, are highly processed.[7] If you want fresh orange juice, buy the oranges and squeeze them yourself. Better yet, just eat the whole orange. Most of the fiber in an orange is in the membranes that surround the orange segments. Eating whole fruit will still quench your thirst and your intestines will be healthier for it.

Herbal teas are also good beverages. Choose teas that contain herbs such as chamomile, passionflower, and/or valerian root for their added calming benefits. Many herbal teas contain caffeine, so make sure the label states that the tea is caffeine free or is marked "no caffeine."

Raw honey, pure maple syrup, and stevia are the best sweetener alternatives for HFCS and aspartame, because they have low-glycemic indexes and don't block leptin. Except for stevia, however, they are all high in calories. Stevia is a very sweet-tasting herb, so a little goes a long way. Stevia can be bitter when used in large amounts; many people use it with another sweetener, such as honey, in baking. Trader Joe's has a powdered version (with lactose added to boost volume) that is easier to use than the pure forms. Be careful when purchasing other brands. Some large food manufacturers have added sugar and artificial ingredients.

You should have your glucose levels checked annually, especially if diabetes tends to run in your family. There are two tests. One is for fasting glucose and the other measures hemoglobin A1c. A normal fasting glucose is considered to be 70 to 99 mg/dl. A blood sugar level from 100 to 125 mg/dl is considered prediabetes and 125 mg/dl or over may indicate diabetes. Before 1997, diabetes was not diagnosed below a level of 140 mg/dl; today's lower level allows better control of diabetes sooner. Those in the 126 to 140 mg/dl range should consider using diet and exercise to manage blood sugar before agreeing to take drugs. Just make sure you have your glucose levels monitored frequently.

The hemoglobin A1c test averages one's blood sugar over two to three months. Hemoglobin, found in red blood cells, carries oxygen throughout the body. When blood sugar is too high, sugar builds up in the blood and glycates, or combines, with hemoglobin. For people without diabetes, the normal range for the hemoglobin A1c test is less than 5.7 percent. Hemoglobin A1c levels from 5.7 to 6.4 percent are considered elevated or prediabetic, and levels of 6.5 percent or higher indicate diabetes. The higher the hemoglobin A1c, the higher the risk of develop-ing complications related to diabetes.

If you are at high risk for diabetes, your doctor will likely recommend both the fasting glucose and the hemoglobin A1c tests. Is it possible to take the fasting glucose and the hemoglobin A1c and receive different results? In other words, can your fasting glucose indicate diabetes while your hemoglobin A1c test indicate normal or vice versa? Yes, the hemo-globin A1c can vary up to 0.5 percent. If this is the case, your doctor should repeat the tests before making a diagnosis.

Lifestyle Choices

NR6

Reduce Stress

Don't keep up with the Joneses. Drag them down to your level. It's cheaper.

~QUENTIN CRISP

MANY HEALTH EXPERTS believe that chronic stress is the cause of most, if not all, disease and illness. The only difference is how stress manifests itself in each body, because we are all born with different genetics, immune systems, strengths, and weaknesses. The human body is made to endure severe and short-lived stress—i.e., acute stress—but does not do as well with chronic stress. Chronic stress is less severe but is persistent and long-lived, lasting months or even years.

Acute stress frequently results in acute illnesses, and chronic stress frequently results in chronic illnesses. The flu is an acute illness that can strike during acute stress, such as studying for finals. The immune system temporarily weakens, making one more susceptible to whatever may be going around. Frequent migraine headaches, backaches, depression, diabetes, and tremors are chronic conditions; they can last months and years. These conditions may result from chronic stress. Working in an unsatisfying job, being in a bad relationship, and dealing with ongoing financial problems are examples of chronic stress.

The brain responds to stress by releasing adrenocorticotropic hormone (ACTH). ACTH stimulates the adrenals to produce the hormones cortisol, epinephrine, and norepinephrine. Epinephrine and norepinephrine, also known as adrenaline, increase blood pressure, constrict blood vessels, and make the heart race, preparing the body for fight-or-flight response. Heightened cortisol levels can have a neurotoxic effect over time and have been linked to accelerated brain aging and short-term memory loss.[1]

Frequently, the few years prior to the development of a chronic condition holds many clues. The stress of a tragic or traumatic event that is difficult to get over, working in a bad job, or staying in a relationship that has gone sour can manifest itself in many ways, mentally and physically. Stress and depression are closely related. We usually become depressed and feel hopeless when we are unable to resolve stressful situations, especially when we are going through them alone. Confiding in a friend, talking to a pastor, or visiting a therapist can make all the difference in the world.

Sometimes "good" stress can get out of hand too. In this high-tech, multitasking, and fast-paced world, many people have high stress levels, but often feel they are "managing" them just fine. They don't realize how much stress they are enduring until they take a vacation or are forced to stop due to an illness. For the most part, books on managing time and stress are useless. Someone who has a problem managing their time probably has too much going on. The best way to manage stress is to reduce it. Evaluate all areas of your life, including relationships, career, finances, and health. Start with an area that causes the most unhappiness and make a change. If you hate your job, look for a new one or investigate a new career. If you have financial problems, track your spending, cut where you can, and budget. If you owe debtors, call them and work out a plan. Sometimes just making that first step toward change can alleviate stress and depression.

If you are depressed and don't know why, get your thyroid hormones and vitamin B12 levels checked. Low thyroid and low vitamin B12 levels can cause anxiety and symptoms of depression. Low vitamin B12 levels can also contribute to memory loss and other neurological problems, if prolonged.

The bottom line is that chronic stress may not be the cause of your tremors, but it can certainly make them worse. Below is a list of natural and effective ways to reduce stress and lift your mood without drugs.

- **Exercise.** This is the number-one way to reduce stress and depression. Exercise has many benefits. It increases endorphins (feel-good hormones), burns calories, improves self-esteem, increases strength, stimulates neuron growth, and reduces anxiety, stress, and depression. You only need a good pair of walking shoes. Walking for 30 minutes every day can do wonders for improving mood and lowering stress levels. Walking in the morning sun is even better—a new study claims that exposure to morning sun increases metabolism. Other great outdoor activities are biking, skating, and even yoga. Exercising outside in the winter helps build the immune system. If that is not practical, then use yoga or aerobics DVDs, or buy a treadmill and some dumbbells. The local health club may also offer seasonal memberships. (See Appendix C for more information on the importance of exercise.)
- **Get good-quality sleep.** Lack of sleep can cause many symptoms, including anxiety, irritability, and depression if prolonged. Insufficient sleep can also trigger or worsen tremors. For the best-quality sleep, get to bed at the same time every night, and wake up at the same time every morning. Drink an herbal tea in the evening with nerve-calming ingredients such as chamomile, valerian, skullcap, hops, or passionflower to help unwind. Melatonin, the sleep hormone, can also help induce sleep. Start with 0.3 mg (300 mcg), 30 to 60 minutes before going to bed. Increase dose slowly for best sleep.
- **Reduce stressful activities.** Watching television, especially news, reality, and crime shows, can increase cortisol levels. The average

American watches more than 5 hours of it per day—over 35 hours a week. That equates to 75 full days a year! The average person who lives to age 80 will have spent over 16 years watching TV. It robs time from other activities and family, increases stress levels, and reduces savings by convincing us to buy things we don't need. Studies have shown that more TV is correlated with higher BMI and depression levels and lower education levels. Reduce your TV watching to an hour per day and get about 25 percent of your life back. Watch comedy shows instead of news and crime shows—laughter reduces stress and depression.

- **Stop drinking.** Alcohol causes fatigue and is a known depressant. It may help stop tremors in the short term, but used long term, alcohol can be addicting.

- **Avoid stimulating drinks and foods.** To keep calm throughout the day, stay away from coffee, sodas, cocoa, caffeinated teas, red meats, processed meats, and sugary snacks. Wheat products can also be stimulating, so avoid them, especially a few hours before bedtime.

- **Take antistress supplements.** Omega-3 fatty acids, B-complex and C vitamins, the minerals magnesium and zinc, and 5-HTP (5-hydroxytryptophan) all help in reducing stress and depression. Deficiency of omega-3 fatty acids is associated with depression. B-complex and C vitamins are natural antistress supplements. Magnesium helps relax nerves and reduce tremors. According to studies, people with depression are often deficient in zinc. Other symptoms of a zinc deficiency are a diminished sense of taste or smell and a lack of appetite. The body naturally converts the neurotransmitter 5-HTP to serotonin, an important hormone for regulating mood and suppressing appetite. However, 5-HTP should not be taken with antidepressant drugs—both increase serotonin levels, which can cause serotonin syndrome, a potentially life-threatening condition.

- **Get a dog.** Studies have shown that people with dogs have lower blood pressure and stress levels overall. Unconditional love and that happy greeting are probably the reason. Taking your dog for a walk in the morning sun will make you happy, increase vitamin D, and help you stay trim. Dogs are also great for meeting people. Not many can resist these lovable creatures.

- **Have fun.** Find an enjoyable activity or hobby and plan on engaging in it at least once a week. Everyone needs something to look forward to.
- **Help others.** Helping others takes our minds off our own problems, especially if we serve the less fortunate.
- **Get a massage.** When performed properly, massage can aid in the healing process by stimulating circulation of immune-system cells, increasing blood flow, soothing tense muscles and joints, inhibiting neurological excitability, increasing flexibility, reducing pain and swelling, lowering blood pressure, and reducing stress and anxiety. Touching the skin lowers the stress hormone cortisol, promoting an increased sense of emotional well-being. However, those with a fever or bruises should avoid any touch therapy until well. Those with blood-clotting problems, cancer, tumors, or an unstable heart condition should get approval from their doctor. Use a licensed massage therapist who is experienced in working with these conditions.

NR7

Get Quality Sleep

*Never under any circumstances take a sleeping pill and a
laxative on the same night.*

~Dave Barry

IN THIS CRAZY, fast-paced world, more and more people are having difficulty getting a good night's sleep. Sleep is important for forming new
memories, making decisions, boosting creativity, clearing out toxins, and
storing and remembering information related to physical tasks. During
sleep, the body builds bone, the pancreas breaks down sugar from the
diet, skin cells churn out growth factors to repair damage and maintain
elasticity, muscles repair tears and injuries, and brain nerve cells dis-
card toxins.[1] A recent study linked sleeping difficulties with a more rapid
decline in brain volume in widespread brain regions.[2]

Lack of sleep can decrease immunity and cause symptoms of anxiety, confusion, depression, forgetfulness, irritability, stress, and *tremors.*
Chronic insomnia is associated with many serious medical conditions,
including diabetes, heart disease, chronic pain, obesity, musculoskeletal

problems, psychiatric disorders, and increased risk of Alzheimer's disease (AD).

According to Dr. Maiken Nedergard at the University of Rochester, certain cells in the brain (glial cells) turn very active when the body sleeps. During the day, glial cells support neurons but cannot conduct electrical impulses themselves. Nedergard found in clinical trials with mice that glial cells slow the brain's electrical activity during sleep, causing neurons to fire in a more synchronized way instead of haphazardly. This lulls nerves into a state of quiet, allowing REM sleep to occur. At the same time, the brain's cells shrink, making way for the brain and spinal cord's fluid to slosh back and forth between them to flush out garbage and toxins.[3] Inadequate sleep means that glial cells can't do their job efficiently. This can lead to neurodegenerative brain disorders later in life. Our brains all have amyloid protein, but in AD, the plaque overtakes healthy brain cells until enough die to cause memory loss.

The most important element of a restful sleep is producing the hormone melatonin. It is not only the body's sleep hormone, it is a powerful antioxidant, anti-inflammatory, and immune-system booster. One study of 10 individuals, with mild cognitive impairment, who took melatonin for 10 consecutive days benefited with improved sleep, memory, and mood, thus suggesting that a restful sleep via increased melatonin may be able to help and prevent AD and dementia.[4] The study might also suggest that quality sleep may improve other neurological conditions, such as ET. Melatonin can be increased naturally by following these tips:

1. **Go to bed before 11:00 p.m. regularly, and get seven to nine hours of sleep.**

   Melatonin production is highest before 11:00 p.m., so a regular sleep schedule is important. Staying up past midnight on weekends makes it difficult to get up early during the week. By the time the body adjusts to the early hours, it is the weekend again. To determine how many hours of sleep you need, go to bed at the same time every night for a couple of weeks (perhaps when you are on vacation or holiday), and do not use an alarm clock to wake up. You may sleep longer the first few nights to catch up on any sleep deprivation that you've accumulated. If you continue going to bed at the same time and allow your body to wake up naturally, you will eventually notice a pattern develop, probably between seven and nine hours of sleep each night.

2. **Do not eat or exercise within two hours of bedtime.**
   If the body is busy digesting food, it can't relax. In addition, it takes hours after exercise for the body to cool down enough to sleep.

3. **Plan the next day on paper.**
   Plan the next day before going to bed. Write down what's on your mind so you won't toss and turn all night thinking about what you need to get done. Keep a pen and paper beside your bed for when you wake in the middle of the night with something on your mind. Write it down and you'll quickly fall back to sleep.

4. **Sleep in complete darkness.**
   Stay away from alarm clocks with lights that stay on all night or anything with a pin light. Studies have shown that even pin lights can keep you from falling into a deep and restful sleep. The light tricks the body into believing it is daytime, preventing melatonin levels from rising.

5. **Add white noise to drown out annoying sounds.**
   If you live in a noisy neighborhood, buy a white-noise machine to block out sounds that keep you awake. Place the machine at least five feet from your bed to prevent electromagnetic energy from reaching you, because electromagnetic frequencies are stimulating. Ceiling fans are great for white noise, and they save on energy in both summer and winter.

6. **Do not drink alcoholic or caffeinated beverages.**
   A nightcap can help you fall asleep, but you are more likely to wake in the middle of the night. Drinking caffeinated beverages, especially in the afternoon, can keep your body stimulated into the evening. Besides, alcohol and caffeine can make tremors worse.

7. **Buy a comfortable mattress.**

   If your mattress is too soft, hard, or old, replace it. One-third of life is spent in bed, so splurge on a comfortable mattress, bedding, and nightwear.

8. **Lower the temperature in the bedroom.**

   Cool air is better for sleeping. Your room should be no warmer than 68 to 70 degrees at night. It is better to throw on covers than to sleep in a stuffy room. In the summer, use a fan and open windows if your bedroom is on the second floor and you live in a safe area. There are security latches available for windows to prevent them from opening wide enough for anyone to enter. Locks on the gates of a fenced-in backyard can provide extra security.

9. **Stretch before bedtime.**

   Ten minutes of stretching or easy yoga poses can help unwind and relax muscles.

10. **Shut off the electronics at least two hours before bedtime.**

    Internet searching, video games, talking or texting on the phone, reading, and television stimulate the brains of most people. The effect can last for hours after stopping the activity. Some people find reading and watching TV before bed relaxing. Read from actual books or basic black-and-white e-readers with the Wi-Fi disabled. The light from self-luminous tablets was found to suppress melatonin production after two hours of use.[5] Watch only happy, funny, or relaxing TV programs before bed (and set a timer to avoid being startled awake in the middle of the night by the bathroom scene in the movie *Psycho*. Trust me on this one).

11. **Resolve emotional issues.**

    Unresolved emotional issues can keep most people from deep sleep. Make a promise to yourself that you'll resolve them. If you are angry at someone from your past that you'll never see again, forgive them in a letter and then shred or burn it. Talking to a trusted friend, minister, pastor, or visiting a psychologist or licensed family therapist can be very helpful.

12. Drink herbal teas to relax.

Teas with the herbs valerian, chamomile, passionflower, and fever-few work well for relaxing mind and body. These herbs can also be taken in supplement form. See NR20 for more information.

13. Take supplements to aid sleep.

Niacin, vitamin B6, and magnesium help increase melatonin levels and are important for reducing tremors. L-theanine, GABA, melatonin, 5-HTP, and the herbs passionflower and valerian are also helpful for inducing restful sleep. 5-HTP can be more helpful for those with insomnia and depression because it supports the production of serotonin, which the body converts to melatonin if needed. Many sleep-formula supplements contain a combination of these substances. (As mentioned in NR6, 5-HTP should never be taken with antidepressants.)

14. Check hormone levels.

Low estrogen and progesterone levels are associated with poor sleep. If you are a woman who has always slept well until reaching your 40s or 50s, your levels of these hormones may be low.

Certain drugs, such as calcium blockers, can lower melatonin production. Check with your doctor if you are taking these or any other medications that may lower melatonin. You may need additional melatonin to get a restful night's sleep.

If the above recommendations don't help you get a good night's sleep, you may have a sleep disorder. The most common of these are night terrors, restless-leg syndrome, sleepwalking, and sleep apnea. Night terrors are different from nightmares in that the affected person wakes up in the middle of the night screaming in terror. Unlike with nightmares, it is almost impossible to wake someone having a night terror. Night terrors are more common in children than adults, but they can happen to anyone. Factors that can contribute are lack of sleep, anxiety, fear of the dark, fever (in children), restless legs, sleep apnea, and low magnesium. Magnesium is also the most important supplement for restless legs. Take at least 300 mg before bed.

Sleepwalking is more common among children than adults, but it can affect anyone. It can be triggered by chaotic sleep schedules, stress disorders, fever, drinking alcohol, sleep apnea, magnesium deficiency, and certain sleep medications. Keeping a regular sleep schedule, avoiding alcohol, reducing stress, and taking magnesium are especially important for preventing sleepwalking.

Sleep apnea is characterized by pauses in breathing or instances of shallow or infrequent breathing during sleep. Each pause in breathing, called an apnea, can last several seconds to several minutes. They can occur hundreds of times per sleeping event. When breathing pauses, carbon dioxide builds up in the bloodstream. When the blood levels of carbon dioxide become high, the brain signals the person to wake and breathe in air. After oxygen is restored, the person falls asleep again.

Sleep apnea can affect anyone, but those at the highest risk are overweight, male, over the age of 40, have a family history, smoke, or have GERD. Sleep apnea deprives the brain of oxygen. Insufficient oxygen results in brain-cell death and memory loss. In one study of elderly women with sleep apnea but without dementia, researchers found that the women had a 44 percent increased risk of developing mild cognitive impairment or dementia than women without sleep apnea.[6] Those with sleep apnea also have increased risk of depression, diabetes, heart problems, high blood pressure, neurological disease, and stroke.

If you suspect you have sleep apnea and are overweight or smoke, losing weight or quitting smoking is crucial. However, due to the seriousness of the risks associated with sleep apnea, a sleep specialist should evaluate you. Several nonsurgical and drugless treatments are available, but surgery can help if other treatments fail or the sleep apnea is caused by a biological reason that only surgery can correct.

NR8

Balance Hormones

*My father invented a cure for which there was no disease
and unfortunately my mother caught it and died of it.*

~VICTOR BORGE

HORMONES ARE THE body's chemical messengers. They travel in the
bloodstream to tissues and organs. They work slowly over time and
affect many processes, including growth and development, metabolism,
mood, reproduction, and sexual function. Endocrine glands make hormones. The major endocrine glands are the adrenal glands, hypothalamus, pancreas, pineal, pituitary, thymus, and thyroid. In addition, men
produce hormones in their testes, and women produce them in their
ovaries.

Endocrine diseases represent some of the most common medical disorders in later life. They are associated with increased risk for dementia,
diabetes, infertility, thyroid problems, *tremors*, weight gain or loss, and
many more. Hormones are powerful. It takes only a tiny amount to cause
big changes in cells or even your whole body. Too much or too little of a

certain hormone can be serious. This is why balanced hormones are critical for optimum health. Laboratory tests can measure the hormone levels in the blood, saliva, or urine.

Except for vitamin D, which is obtained from direct sunlight absorbed by the skin or from supplements, hormones are produced by several glands in the body. Here, the focus is on the hormone-producing glands or organs that are most likely to cause symptoms of shaking if they do not function properly. These include the adrenal glands, hypothalamus, ovaries, pancreas, pineal, and thyroid. Testosterone deficiency is unlikely to cause tremors, but men of "a certain age" should be tested at their annual checkups. Low testosterone levels can contribute to many other problems, including fatigue, low libido, and weight gain.

Adrenal glands

The adrenal glands sit on top of the kidneys in the deepest part of the abdomen and release hormones in response to stress. These hormones are cortisol, adrenaline (also called epinephrine), and noradrenaline (also called norepinephrine). The adrenal glands also produce androgen hormones and aldosterone. Androgen hormones, mainly produced in the testes, are male sex hormones responsible for typical male physical characteristics. Aldosterone is a hormone that helps regulate water and salt in the body.

Cortisol, the main stress hormone, regulates many functions in the body related to stress including blood sugar levels, immunity, healing, energy, blood pressure, and inflammation. Too much stress depletes cortisol. Prolonged levels of cortisol in the bloodstream can impair its job, resulting in increased blood sugar levels, lower immunity, slower healing, depleted energy, higher blood pressure, and chronic inflammation.

A tumor on the adrenal gland can cause it to produce too much adrenaline or noradrenaline. One of the symptoms is hand tremors. Other symptoms are abdominal pain, anxiety, blurred vision, blood sugar variations, constipation, headaches, high blood sugar, pale skin, panic attacks, rapid heart rate, sweating, and weight loss.

Hypothalamus

The hypothalamus gland is about the size of a pea and is located just below the thalamus and above the brain stem. Its main functions are to control body temperature, hunger, thirst, blood pressure, levels of hormones in circulation, and secretion of melatonin for sleep. It also controls changes in cortisol. The hypothalamus controls the pituitary gland, mostly in its response to stress. The pituitary gland controls the adrenal glands, thyroid gland, female ovaries, and male testes.

The hormones produced by the hypothalamus gland include oxytocin and antidiuretic hormones. Oxytocin stimulates contraction of the uterus during childbirth and aids in breastfeeding. Antidiuretic hormones aid the reabsorption of water in the kidneys. Without antidiuretic hormones, thirst and urination become excessive.

Although problems with the hypothalamus gland do not directly cause shaking or affect ET, its major role in controlling other hormone levels may do so indirectly. For instance, insomnia from low melatonin levels or an increase in cortisol levels can trigger tremors.

Brain injury, benign tumor, infection, radiation, and surgery are some causes of hypothalamus dysfunction. Common symptoms related to dysfunction of this gland include cold intolerance, constipation, depression, dizziness, fatigue, hair or skin changes, loss of body hair and muscle in men, mental slowing, weakness, and weight gain. Headaches and vision loss are symptoms of a tumor. Having any of these symptoms does not guarantee that a person has hypothalamus dysfunction, as these are all common symptoms for many conditions. However, if you have several of these symptoms, it may be wise to get examined to rule out any problems with the hypothalamus.

Ovaries

Low levels of female sex hormones can cause tremors. The ovaries produce the female sex hormones estrogen and progesterone, in addition to a small amount of testosterone. In women, testosterone is also produced by the adrenal glands. Estrogen can drop 40 to 60 percent by the time a woman reaches menopause. Progesterone levels can drop even lower.

Estrogen stimulates the growth of new neurons and connections and improves blood circulation, mood, memory, and clear thinking. Many women joke about having "senior moments" in their 40s, but declining estrogen levels are nothing to joke about. Estrogen deficiency can cause brain fog, depression, short-term memory loss, low libido, hot flashes, night sweats, moodiness, trouble sleeping, and dry hair, nails, and skin.

Progesterone helps the body use fat for energy, reduce water weight, normalize sleep patterns, facilitate thyroid-hormone function, promote bone production, and normalize blood-sugar levels. Deficiency of progesterone is linked to belly fat, bloating, insomnia, and low blood sugar.

Most women start to experience drops in hormone levels as early as their 30s. Is conventional hormone replacement therapy (HRT) the answer? Some studies have linked HRT with breast cancer, heart disease, and blood clots. However, the estrogen and progesterone used in these studies were synthetic. Unlike synthetic hormones, natural transdermal creams, made from plant sources, are not metabolized by the liver, making them much safer if used properly. Progesterone is safer to take than estrogen by itself because it is a precursor to cortisol, estrogen, and testosterone—meaning that these hormones can be made or converted from progesterone if the body needs them. On the other hand, estrogen should *always* be taken with progesterone to avoid risk of estrogen dominance, which is linked to cancer.

Natural progesterone creams are available without a prescription, but they come in stock formulations, so you may need to experiment with them for a while to get the right dosage. This is fine short term, but eventually, lab tests should be performed, especially if you are having difficulty determining the proper dosage. Saliva, urine, or blood tests can help determine the levels of hormones the body needs, though blood tests are not as accurate as urine and saliva tests. Since hormone levels in the body change continuously, tests should be updated every 6 to 12 months. Natural estrogen creams are also available, but proper dosage should be determined with labs tests. As mentioned earlier, estrogen should be balanced with progesterone to reduce risk of estrogen dominance.

Before resorting to HRT, there are many things that can be done to help balance hormones in both men and women. Following a healthy diet, exercising, getting quality sleep, and avoiding endocrine disruptors are all very important for keeping hormones balanced. Keeping optimal levels of vitamin D and getting plenty of omega-3 EFAs and saturated fats are essential for hormone metabolism. Herbs such as maca root (also referred to as Peruvian ginseng) can also help balance hormones in men and women. Maca root has been used by the native Andean people for centuries to increase stamina and fertility. In addition, maca root is used for menopausal symptoms, premenstrual syndrome, sexual dysfunction, and as an aphrodisiac.

Pancreas

The pancreas is a large organ in the abdomen located near the stomach and bowel. It produces digestive enzymes to aid in the breakdown and digestion of food. The pancreas also produces the hormone insulin, which controls blood sugar levels.

Insulin is important for keeping blood sugar levels from fluctuating too much. One of the symptoms of low blood sugar, or hypoglycemia, is shaking. Other symptoms include anxiety, confusion, dizziness, fatigue, and hunger. Hypoglycemia can lead to insulin resistance and type 2 diabetes. Anyone who has these symptoms or is over 30 years of age should have their glucose levels checked.

Pineal Gland

The pineal gland is located deep in the brain between the right and left lobes, just above the thalamus. It works in harmony with the hypothalamus gland, directing the body's thirst, hunger, sexual desire, and the biological clock that determines our aging process.

The pineal gland produces melatonin. A cyst or tumor on the pineal gland can impair melatonin production. Symptoms of pineal dysfunction to look for include dizziness, fatigue, hearing and speech problems, insomnia, nausea, and vomiting. Low melatonin levels do not cause tremors; however, chronic lack of sleep due to low melatonin levels may worsen existing ones.

Thyroid

The thyroid is butterfly-shaped, with two lobes, and is located just below the Adam's apple in the neck. The thyroid gland produces hormones that regulate metabolic rate, heart and digestive function, bone maintenance, muscle control, and brain development. The thyroid produces thyroid hormones and calcitonin, which plays a role in regulating calcium levels in the body.

The thyroid can become underactive (hypothyroidism) or overactive (hyperthyroidism). Hypothyroidism is characterized by brain fog, brittle nails, chronic sinusitis, constipation, cold intolerance, depression, dry and thinning hair, dry skin, fatigue, muscle cramps, mild cognitive impairment, and weight gain. Hypothyroidism can be treated with natural or synthetic medicine.

One of the symptoms of hyperthyroidism is shaking, including hand tremors. Other signs of hyperthyroidism include brittle hair, irritability, insomnia, nervousness, panic or anxiety disorders, rapid heartbeat, and weight loss. For older women, thyroid problems also double the risk of developing Alzheimer's disease.[1] Hyperthyroidism can be treated with medication, but it has very undesirable side effects. An overactive thyroid can be treated naturally by avoiding excitotoxins and other stimulants, eating a healthy diet, using calming herbs, and getting a good night's sleep.

Many people have undiagnosed thyroid problems because symptoms can be vague or mimic other conditions. Have your thyroid checked annually if you are over the age of 40 or more often if you have symptoms related to thyroid-hormone imbalances. Insurance usually covers these tests.

NR9

Avoid Tremor-Inducing Drugs

*You and your doctor have been screwed into believing
every symptom is a deficiency of some drug or surgery. You've been led to believe you have no control,
when in truth you're the one who must take control.
Unfortunately, the modus operandi in medicine is to find
a drug to turn off the damaged part that is producing
symptoms.*

~Sherry A. Rogers

DRUG-INDUCED TREMORS ARE common and often resemble ET. Medications
that cause tremors can also increase intensity of existing tremors, or
they can create tremors that imitate the resting tremors of Parkinson's
disease. If your tremors developed or increased in severity after starting
a medication, don't assume it is ET or that the condition is progressing.
See your doctor immediately.

Before purchasing any new prescription drug, always ask the pharmacist for the packaging insert so you can check the list of side effects

yourself. Don't count on your doctor to know all the side effects of a particular drug. If possible, avoid newly-marketed drugs for which there is no generic available. In recent years, the FDA has allowed shorter test periods before a drug hits the market, and serious side effects often don't show up until several years later. In addition to being very risky, new drugs are very expensive.

Work with a healthcare practitioner to reduce your dependency on medications. Taking one drug frequently results in the taking of another to alleviate the side effects of the first. Plus, drugs only cover up the symptoms and don't get to the root of the problem. They can be helpful in the short term while working to find a healthier alternative, but drugs should seldom be a long-term solution. Never abruptly stop or reduce dosage of prescription drugs without your doctor's consent and/or monitoring. Some drugs can produce serious symptoms if reduced too quickly. If your doctor refuses to work with you, find one that will, or go to an alternative healthcare practitioner.

Discussed below are medications commonly found to cause or worsen tremors along with natural alternatives. This is not a complete list of drugs, as new side effects are always being reported, and new drugs are always entering the marketplace. Any side effects mentioned were obtained from www.drugs.com (with permission).

Asthma medications

Asthma is a condition in which the airways narrow and swell, making breathing difficult. Symptoms of asthma, depending on severity, include coughing, wheezing, and shortness of breath. Symptoms can be triggered by allergies, exercise, or air pollutants. Medications used to control asthma long term are corticosteroids (inhaled, oral, and IV), leukotriene modifiers, short- and long-acting beta agonists, combination inhalers, and theophylline. All of these medications can cause tremors. Albuterol and levalbuterol are short-acting beta agonists. Montelukast (Singulair), zafirlukast (Accolate), and zileuton (Zyflo) are leukotriene modifiers. Combination inhalers include a corticosteroid and a leukotriene modifier.

Asthma medications can be a life saver for those with severe symptoms, so there are not many other options, at least initially. Allergy shots (immunotherapy) can work wonders, but they take time and money. Immunotherapy works by gradually reducing immune system reactions to specific allergens. This process usually takes three to five years. As a child, I had moderate to severe asthma. Allergy shots were a life saver for me.

Natural ways to reduce asthma symptoms are by exercising with caution, avoiding air pollutants, and eliminating airborne and food allergens as much as possible. Exercising can help strengthen the lungs. Start by walking every day and increase the time and pace slowly. Air pollution can worsen asthma symptoms. Stay inside when outdoor air pollution is at moderate to high levels. To reduce indoor air pollution, keep humidity levels low to prevent mold growth. Reduce exposure to household chemicals by cleaning regularly with natural products, encasing mattresses and pillows with dust proof covers, and replacing wall-to-wall carpeting with hardwood or linoleum flooring. There's more on household chemicals in NR12. In addition, during pollen season, keep windows closed and use air conditioning to reduce airborne allergens. To reduce food allergens, avoid foods that cause allergy symptoms—itchy throat, hives, abdominal pain, nausea, diarrhea, vomiting, dizziness, migraine, wheezing, and trouble breathing—right after eating. Some of these symptoms can also be indicative of other conditions, such as celiac disease or IBS, so it is important to see a doctor for testing. Although any food can cause an allergic reaction, the most common food allergens are dairy, eggs, wheat, fish, shellfish, soy, peanuts, and tree nuts.

Supplements helpful in blocking histamine and inflammation are quercetin and vitamin C with bioflavonoids. During allergy season, take 400 mg of quercetin twice a day—one in the morning and one in the evening. Take 500 to 2,000 mg of vitamin C a day, depending on symptoms. Spread doses in excess of 500 mg evenly throughout the day—for example, take 500 mg at every meal and at bedtime. Reduce dosage of vitamin C if stools become loose.

Antidepressants

These medications are used to relieve severe anxiety, panic attacks, depression, and OCD (obsessive-compulsive disorder). SSRIs (selective reuptake inhibitors) and tricyclic antidepressants are the two types that commonly cause tremors. SSRIs are the mostly widely prescribed antidepressants. They include citalopram (Celexa), escitalopram (Lexapro), fluoxetine (Prozac), fluvoxamine (Luvox), fluvoxamine CR (Luvox CR), paroxetine (Paxil), paroxetine CR (Paxil CR), and sertraline (Zoloft). Tricyclic antidepressants include amitriptyline (Elavil), amoxapine, desipramine (Norpramin), doxepine (Sinequan), imipramine (Tofranil), nortriptyline (Pamelor), protriptyline (Vivactil), and trimipramine (Surmontil).

Common side effects of these antidepressants are numerous, including dizziness, dry mouth, insomnia, sexual dysfunction, *tremors*, and weight gain. In some studies, antidepressants worked only slightly better than a placebo. This could mean that depression in most people subsides whether or not they take a drug. Never abruptly stop taking antidepressants; they have some of the worse withdrawal symptoms of any drugs. Your doctor can develop a plan to help wean you off them.

There are many natural ways to treat depression. First, get your thyroid and vitamin B12 levels checked. Low thyroid and vitamin B12 levels can cause anxiety and symptoms of depression. Proven ways to alleviate depression include several or all of the following: exercise, sunshine, a wholesome diet free of artificial ingredients and junk food, lifestyle changes to reduce stress, antistress supplements (see NR6), massage therapy, and talking to someone about your problems.

Calcium-channel blockers (CCBs)

CCBs, or calcium antagonists, are used in the treatment of high blood pressure (HBP), chest pain (angina), and irregular heartbeats (arrhythmia). Calcium goes through tiny "channels" into the heart muscle cells and smooth muscle cells of the arteries, which causes arteries to contract, or narrow. CCBs work by reducing the amount of calcium that goes through these tiny "channels," causing the heart muscles and arteries to relax, allowing blood to flow more smoothly. This helps lower blood pressure, alleviate angina, or control arrhythmia. Commonly prescribed CCBs that can cause shaking include amlodipine (Norvasc), nifedipine (Adalat, Procardia), nicardipine (Cardene), and verapamil (Calan, Isoptin, and Verelan). There are many more CCBs available so if yours was not mentioned, check www.drugs.com for the list of side effects.

The Dietary Approaches to Stop Hypertension (DASH) diet has been shown to reduce HBP without the use of drugs. It includes plenty of fruits, vegetables, whole grains, fish, poultry, nuts, and fat-free or low-fat dairy. Fats, red meats, sweets, and sugary beverages are restricted. The DASH diet is fine except for the exclusion of coconut oil and the inclusion of vegetable oils and fat-free or low-fat dairy. As discussed in NR3, there are several recent studies showing no significant evidence that saturated fat in the diet is linked to increased risk of cardiovascular disease. Coconut oil, extra virgin olive oil, and butter are much healthier than vegetable oils. There is also little evidence that milk or other dairy products benefit bones. However, whole-milk, plain yogurt and aged or raw cheese have the benefits of probiotics, but even these should be consumed in moderation. Some research shows that consuming too much dairy may contribute to the risk of prostate and ovarian cancers, autoimmune diseases, and some childhood ailments.[1] Preferably, dairy products should come from grass-fed, pasture-raised cows or goats. Almond, cashew, and organic soy milks are acceptable alternatives for cow's milk.

Exercise is also extremely important for lowering blood pressure or preventing HBP. Brisk walking for 30 minutes, 5 times per week, is sufficient. Researchers have found that walking 10 minutes, 3 times per day, is even more effective than one 30-minute session.[2] See Appendix C for more information on exercise.

The best supplements to take for HBP are magnesium, potassium, omega-3 EFAs, CoQ10, garlic, fiber, and the herb hawthorn. Those with kidney disorders should check with their doctor before taking potassium.

CNS Stimulants

CNS stimulants are substances that speed up brain and nervous system functions. They are most commonly used to improve attention span, lose weight, and treat asthma, migraine headaches, and pain.

Amphetamines are CNS stimulants that are highly addictive and therefore widely abused by people in professional sports, the entertainment industry, executive positions, and those who struggle to lose weight, including professional models. Many medications contain amphetamine components, including some used to treat ADHD (attention deficit hyperactivity disorder), colds, narcolepsy, pain, and weight gain. Abuse of these drugs causes nervous system disorders and cardiovascular fatalities. All CNS stimulants, legal and illegal, can destroy the nervous system and trigger movement disorders, including tremors. Symptoms are not always reversible after drug withdrawal.

Common over-the-counter medications with amphetamines are cold medications, pain relievers, and diet pills. Prescribed medications include dextroamphetamine (Dexedrine and Adderall), diethylpropion (Tenuate, Tenuate Dospan, Tepanil), phentermine (Adipex-P, Obestin-30, phentermine resin oral), methylphenadate (Ritalin, Concerta, Metadate), and pemoline (Cylert).

Nicotine, found in tobacco products, is another addictive CNS stimulant. Smoking or chewing tobacco can cause shaking and tremors. Besides nicotine, tobacco products contain approximately 2,000 chemicals. These chemicals infuse the brain with free radicals which creates inflammation, eventually resulting in neuron death. According to a 2014 report from the surgeon general, smoking increases risk of type 2 diabetes, cancer, heart disease, and strokes.

Caffeine is another CNS stimulant that is everywhere these days. It is in coffee, tea, sodas, chocolate, and many medications. Common side effects of too much caffeine include anxiety, depression, difficulty sleeping, nausea, restlessness, rapid heart rate, tremors, frequent urination, and vomiting. Caffeine in moderation for anyone without a nervous condition is fine, but not for anyone with ET or other nervous symptom disorders. Caffeine will worsen symptoms. Decaffeinated (decaf) coffee is an option, but most companies use chemical solvents to remove the caffeine. Plus, most decaf coffees still contain a small amount of caffeine (typically two to five milligrams) that can worsen tremors in sensitive individuals. If you can't live without your "cup of joe," look for decaf coffee made with the Swiss Water process by the Swiss Water Decaffeinated Coffee Company. They claim to remove 99.9 percent of the caffeine without chemical solvents.

There are natural ways to treat ADHD, alleviate pain and migraines, and lose weight. To treat ADHD, avoid food dyes, preservatives, artificial ingredients, and foods linked to behavioral disorders such as chocolate, eggs, dairy, and frankenwheat. Increase intake of omega-3 fatty acids. When taken regularly, omega-3 supplements have prompted significant improvements in behavior, attention, and mood in several studies. Other helpful supplements are magnesium, zinc, and phosphatidylserine (PS).

Poor diet and lifestyle choices are the two most common causes of chronic pain and migraine headaches. If your life is very stressful, work on reducing stress and increasing relaxation. Chocolate, dairy products (especially cheese), caffeine, MSG, aspartame, processed meats, nuts (if allergic), frankenwheat, and wine can trigger migraines. People with migraines are found to have lower serum levels of magnesium than those who do not have them. Intravenous (IV) magnesium has been used in the treatment of acute migraines and fibromyalgia. This makes sense given that magnesium is critical for proper nerve and muscle function. Research has also shown that people who experience chronic constipation tend to have more headaches. Magnesium also helps relieve constipation. Other supplements helpful in reducing migraines are riboflavin (vitamin B2), CoQ10, and the herbs butterbur and feverfew. Turmeric, capsaicin (found in chili pepper), SAM-e, MSM, and omega-3 EFAs can also ease pain in arthritis, fibromyalgia, migraines, and other chronic conditions by reducing inflammation. In addition, alternative therapies such as massage and chiropractic can be helpful in reducing chronic pain in some individuals.

If you are overweight, have your levels of thyroid and sex hormones tested to rule out hormonal imbalances. Low thyroid, estrogen, progesterone, or testosterone levels can cause weight gain. Following the recommendations in the *Food Choices* section in Part III and Appendix C: Importance of Exercise is a better way to lose weight and prevent weight gain in the future than taking drugs or following fad or extreme diets.

Ingredients that support weight loss are fiber, MCTs, and citric acid. Fiber is found in plant foods—legumes, nuts, fruits, vegetables, and whole grains, with the highest amounts in legumes and whole grains. MCTs are the only fats that help with weight loss because they are not stored in the body like other fats; coconut oil is the best source. Foods with citric acid speed up the metabolism; oranges, lemons, and berries (except blueberries) are the best sources. Drinking a cup of tea with freshly-squeezed lemon, about 30 minutes before breakfast, will jump start your metabolism.

Chromium picolinate is a popular weight-loss supplement, but it has not been found to be very helpful for losing weight in studies, even at very high doses. Chromium picolinate was found, however, to be effective in balancing blood sugar in those that have diabetes.

Decongestants

Decongestants are used in the treatment of colds and allergies. Common brand-name drugs include Actifed Daytime Allergy, Claritin-D, Dimetapp, NyQuil, Sudafed, Sinustop, and the Triaminic Allergy Congestion offerings. Besides tremors, this class of drugs can also cause memory loss.

To relieve congestion naturally, start by eliminating all dairy and gluten. For cold-related congestion, heat a pot of water and add a few drops of eucalyptus oil. Cover your head with a towel over the pot and breathe in the vapors. Do this two times a day. Eating hot soup with lots of spices helps clear the sinuses as well. Quercetin and vitamin C with bioflavonoids can be helpful for both allergy- and cold-related congestion. For cold symptoms, take 500 mg of vitamin C every four hours and/or 400 mg of quercetin twice a day—one in the morning and one in the evening—until symptoms subside. Reduce dosage of vitamin C if stools become loose. The best food sources of quercetin and vitamin C are apples, berries, citrus fruits, garlic, kale, onions, and peppers, so increase consumption of these as well.

Mood stabilizers

Mood stabilizers, or antipsychotics, are used mainly to treat mood problems associated with schizophrenia and to prevent mania in bipolar disorder. They are also used to stabilize mood and alleviate delusions and hallucinations, including in people with dementia and Alzheimer's disease.

Common antipsychotic drugs include haloperidol (Haldol), chlorpromazine (Thorazine), risperidone (Risperdal), aripiprazole (Abilify), olanzapine (Zyprexa), quetiapine (Seroquel), ziprasidone (Geodon), sulpiride, and lithium. Antipsychotics have some of the most severe side effects of any class of drugs. They include agitation, depression, dizziness, nausea, somnolence, suicidal behavior, *tremors*, vomiting, and weight gain. Less common, but more disturbing, side effects of antipsychotics are congestive heart failure, hallucinations, seizures, uncontrolled movements, parkinsonism, and rhabdomyolysis.

In studies, psychosis has been associated with nutritional deficiencies, especially of magnesium, folic acid, niacin (B3), and vitamin B12. When deficiencies are identified and fixed, amazing results have followed. People with allergies and those who abuse stimulants also have increased risk of psychosis. Lifestyle changes that make huge differences in mood disorders are acupuncture, aromatherapy, exercise, massage therapy, meditation, psychological counseling, sauna therapy, and yoga.

Thyroid hormone replacement

Thyroid hormone replacement is used to improve an underactive thyroid, or hypothyroidism. Too high of a dose can cause shaking. Levothyroxine (Synthroid, Levothroid, Levoxyl, and Unithroid) is the most common drug used to treat hypothyroidism.

The main cause of low thyroid is insufficient iodine, an essential mineral needed for the secretion of thyroid hormone. Some of the causes of iodine deficiency are gluten, heavy metals, endocrine disruptors, and stress.

A significant number of people with thyroid disease also have celiac disease. Going on a gluten-free diet may help improve thyroid function, as well as reduce tremors.

Heavy metals and other toxins can destroy the thyroid gland. Drinking alcohol and smoking can damage the thyroid and trigger or worsen tremors, so avoid these bad habits.

Bromine, a common endocrine disruptor that displaces iodine in the body, is found in pesticides (as methyl bromide), citrus-flavored soft drinks (brominated vegetable oils), medications, flours (as potassium bromate), and flame retardants. Detoxing periodically with a detoxification diet and chelating supplements like chlorella and vitamin C will help keep the thyroid, along with the liver and kidneys, from being overloaded. A good book on how to use diet to detoxify is *The Detox Diet* by Dr. Elson M. Haas.

Last but not least, regular exercise is important for eliminating toxins and normalizing stress hormones that can impair thyroid function. Exercise also stimulates growth of new brain cells, an important consideration for anyone with a neurological condition. See Appendix C for more information.

Supplements that enhance thyroid function are selenium, kelp, vitamin B12, and omega-3 fatty acids. Kelp is a natural source of iodine; just make sure it is free of contaminants and sourced from the Atlantic and not the Pacific Ocean. Norwegian kelp is the best.

Taking a natural hormone replacement like desiccated (dried) thyroid made by Armour or NatureThroid is another option, except for vegetarians and vegans. These supplements, called glandulars, are made from pork-thyroid glands.

Other medications

Certain antianxieties, antibiotics, cancer drugs (thalidomide and cytarabine), and heart medicines (amiodarone, procainamide, and others) can cause tremors. In addition, medications that suppress immune function (cyclosporine and tacrolimus), treat shingles and herpes viruses (acyclovir and vidarabine), and certain medications that help prevent seizures (valproic acid and sodium valproate) can also do the same.

—m—

Note on drug addiction and withdrawal

Withdrawal from alcohol and certain medications such as benzodiazepines (alprazolam, diazepam, lorazepam, and others) can cause tremors, as well as many other unpleasant symptoms. If you are addicted to any drug (legal or illegal), tobacco, or alcohol, join the appropriate support group and find a medical professional who specializes in drug addiction.

NR10

Catch Some Rays

*You have to stay in shape. My grandmother started walk-
ing five miles a day when she was 60. She's 97 today and
we don't know where the hell she is.*

~ELLEN DeGeneres

Most Americans spend the majority of their time indoors. We have office
jobs during the day and electronics to keep us busy at night. When
we do venture out in the sun, we slather on sunscreen for fear of developing skin cancer. Because of this lifestyle, most Americans are deficient in
vitamin D. Ironically, deficiency of vitamin D, or calciferol, can increase risk
of certain cancers.

Vitamin D is classified as a fat-soluble vitamin, but it has properties
of a hormone. It is related structurally to the hormones estrogen and
cortisone. The main function of vitamin D is to help the body absorb calcium and phosphorus, minerals essential for proper bone structure and
strength. Vitamin D has always been associated with prevention of bone
diseases (osteopenia, osteomalacia, and osteoporosis), bone fractures,

rickets, and tooth decay. More recent studies have shown vitamin D to have antidepressant, anti-inflammatory, immune-boosting, and neuro-protective properties. Researchers have linked low or deficient levels of vitamin D to many more chronic conditions, including certain cancers (breast, prostate, and colon), Crohn's disease, hyperthyroidism, hyper-parathyroidism, depression, heart disease, diabetes, cognitive decline, dementia, PD, seasonal affective disorder (SAD), and autoimmune dis-eases such as Grave's disease, Hashimoto's thyroiditis, inflammatory bowel disease (IBD), lupus, MS, rheumatoid arthritis, and type 1 diabetes.

One of the symptoms of hyperthyroidism, including Grave's disease, and hyperparathyroidism is hand tremors. No studies have been per-formed to determine if there is a link between ET and low levels of vita-min D; however, deficiencies are common in PD and MS, two neurological conditions that present tremors as a symptom. Boosting vitamin D levels can help prevent bone diseases, depression, SAD, cognitive decline, PD, autoimmune diseases, and many other conditions. It may also reduce or prevent tremors.

Vitamin D is called the "sunshine" vitamin because human skin manu-factures it when in contact with ultraviolet light from the sun's rays. The energy of the sun's radiation is necessary to create the right chemical reaction that turns the precursor cholesterols into a form of vitamin D the body can use. By the time a person reaches his or her 70s, the precursor to vitamin D generally found in skin diminishes three- or fourfold, making it increasingly difficult to produce enough vitamin D naturally. Serum lev-els of vitamin D can be measured by using the 25-hydroxy vitamin D test. A blood-serum level of vitamin D below 30 ng/ml is considered deficient. An optimum level to aim for is 50 ng/ml.

The sun is the best source of vitamin D. Sun exposure of 20 min-utes, three or four times per week, is sufficient for most people. Enjoyable activities such as gardening, walking, playing tennis, or biking are great ways to absorb rays. After 20 minutes, putting on a chemical-free sun-screen or covering up can help prevent skin aging and skin cancer. Taking the powerful antioxidant astaxanthin can allow up to three times longer exposure to the sun; it prevents sunburn naturally.

Another way to get more vitamin D is to increase consumption of vitamin D-rich foods such as eggs, butter, fish (salmon, sardines, tuna, and herring), and mushrooms (shiitake and chanterelle). Fortified food products like breakfast cereals are enriched with vitamin D; however, their low nutritional value means they are not the best daily choice. Milk has vitamin D, but it is not recommended because of its many health risks. As previously mentioned, there is no significant data to support the claim that the consumption of dairy leads to better bones or improved health. On the contrary, researchers in Sweden found milk correlated with higher mortality in men and women and higher bone fractures in women.[1]

Vitamin D supplementation is a good idea, especially in the winter months for those living in temperate climate zones, those unable to spend time in the sun, and those with neurological conditions like tremors. There are two forms of vitamin D: D2 (ergocalciferol) and D3 (cholecalciferol). Vitamin D2 is made by irradiating yeast or mushrooms. It is used primarily by vegans, vegetarians, and food manufacturers to fortify processed foods. Vitamin D3 is made from lanolin or lichen. Lanolin is the grease from the wool of sheep, and lichen is an organism composed of algae and fungus. Vitamin D3 is also found in cod liver oil. Vitamin D3 is preferred because it converts easily to fully active vitamin D, whereas D2 does not.

Recommendations vary for adults, from 1,000 to 2,000 international units (IU) daily. Those with a known vitamin D deficiency should take doses of 5,000 IU a day or more until levels are back to normal. Prescriptions are usually written for vitamin D2 and in very high amounts—for example, 25,000 IU or more per week to be taken all at once. However, D2 can be toxic in high amounts. Common symptoms of vitamin D toxicity include excessive thirst, diarrhea, weakness, headaches, and bone pain. Symptoms usually decrease and disappear when megadoses are stopped.

Vitamin D works in synergy with calcium, magnesium, and vitamins A and K2. The body can use vitamin D best when it's taken with vitamin A (found in all multivitamins). Vitamin D helps absorb calcium. Vitamins K1 and K2 are important for blood clotting, but vitamin K2 is also critical for keeping bones strong and arteries clear, so it is the preferred form.

Calcium supplements have been associated with increased risk of myocardial infarction.[2] Calcium, not cholesterol, now seems to be the culprit in heart disease. The reason for this, according to Robert Thompson, MD, author of *The Calcium Lie*, is an imbalance of mineral supplements. The average American gets plenty of calcium in fortified foods because food manufacturers believe that calcium supplementation prevents bone loss. However, without sufficient amounts of magnesium and vitamin K2 to transport calcium to bones, it ends up in the arteries and elsewhere, causing calcification. Calcification is the hardening of tissue matter and the main cause of kidney stones. Those who get sufficient calcium in the diet do not need supplementation. Foods rich in calcium are almonds, broccoli, kale, collard greens, edamame, salmon, white beans, and tofu. Foods rich in vitamin K2 are fermented products such as sauerkraut, natto, kefir, and raw cheese. Supplements of vitamin K2 are also available. Vitamin K is a natural blood thinner; those on anticoagulant (blood-thinner) medications should seek their doctor's approval before taking.

Environmental Factors

NR11

Electromagnetic Fields

Radio wave sickness and electromagnetic hypersensitivity are easily preventable and one can only wonder how much longer the insanity of modern governments is going to be allowed to continue in this area.

~STEVEN MAGEE

ALMOST EVERY ADULT, teen, and child in every industrialized country has a cell phone, laptop or tablet, and television. Most households also have cordless phones, wireless printers, game consoles, wireless alarm systems, and smart utility meters, or smart meters. All of these wireless technologies emit electromagnetic fields (EMFs).

Twenty years ago, few people owned cell phones. Now there are more cell phones in the United States than people. The Federal Communications Commission (FCC) determined the safety of wireless devices based on their thermal effects by placing a turned-on cell phone near the head of a mannequin for six minutes. The mannequin's head was filled with liquid. Since the mannequin's temperature did not change more than one degree Celsius after six minutes, the FCC determined cell phones to be safe.[1] This study was flawed on many levels. First, the mannequin was six feet, two inches tall and weighed over 200 pounds, representing only a small fraction of the population and ignoring the potential effects of cell phone use on smaller men, most women, and children. Second, the average use of a cell phone has increased significantly beyond the six minutes used in the study. Third, the study kept the phone one inch from the mannequin's head. Most people put their phones against their ears during calls, and otherwise into a pocket that is against their bodies. Fourth, scientists have found many *nonthermal* effects of using cell phones. In one Swedish study, scientists discovered a significant increase in the risk for brain tumors when cell phone use exceeded 10 years.[2] In another Swedish study, researchers found that brain cancer rates have increased in Norway, Denmark, and parts of Sweden, the first countries to use cell phones. The Swedish researchers also discovered that DNA brain cell damage has an average latency period of over 30 years before increased cancer rates are expected. The results were age-adjusted, showing increased cancer rates in both younger and older age groups.[3] In the United States, cell phone use significantly increased after the release of the iPhone in 2007, about nine years ago. Based on the Swedish research, we may not see an epidemic of brain cancer and neurological conditions until the mid-to-late 2030s. If we do, it will likely include young people in their 30s who started using smart phones and other wireless technologies when they were toddlers.

Other researchers, at Lund University Hospital in Sweden, exposed 32 male and female laboratory rats for two hours to mobile phones. Leakage was found in the blood-brain barrier, and neuronal damage was noted in the cortex, hippocampus, and basal ganglia areas of the brains of the exposed rats.[4] Leakage in the blood-brain barrier allows toxins into the brain, leading to death of brain neurons. What are a few billion fewer brain cells—you have plenty, right?

The FDA, American Cancer Society (ACS), and the World Health Organization (WHO) classify radiation from cell phones as possibly carcinogenic to humans. None of these agencies believe any studies so far prove an absolute link. Even if a definite link is found, will the wireless phone companies, who have billions of dollars of sales at risk, try to cover it up? Does a cover-up already exist?

What about the new smart meters? Electric companies across the United States, Canada, the United Kingdom, and many other countries are installing smart meters at electrifying speed (pun intended). Smart meters have not been studied to see if they cause health problems according to the ACS. So should we believe our utility company when they tell us that smart meters are perfectly safe when studies have not been performed? At one time, most of us thought lead paint, asbestos, and smoking were safe. Many have paid the price with their life for those errors.

Smart meters transmit information to the utility companies throughout the day—from a few times per day to several times per minute or second. If you have a smart meter, every time it transmits, radiation is pulsed throughout your house—more so if you have smart appliances. Then there's the privacy issue. The utility company can read the activity of your appliances. Do you really want others to know when you watch TV, wash your clothes, dry your hair, or do something even more personal—and to sell the information to marketers? The utility companies may tell you that your privacy is protected, but for how long? Smart meters, along with smart appliances, can also be hacked. Isn't worrying about your computer getting hacked enough?

In addition, electrical wiring in many homes is not updated for modern wireless technology. This results in another scary problem; some smart meters explode and catch fire causing major damage to homes.[5] The utility companies don't want to admit the problem because they don't want the responsibility of replacing meters they've spent millions on.

Smart meters negatively affect health, invade privacy, and are a possible fire hazard. They may not be so smart after all.

What about the decrease in bee populations? Experts do not know for sure what is causing the bee population to decrease, but they have a name for it—colony collapse disorder (CCD). This is a critical problem for the food supply, because one in three plants requires pollination from bees to survive. So far, two major changes in the past two decades could be blamed. One is wireless technology, and the other is the increase in herbicides used on plants grown from GM seeds. In studies, mobile phones placed next to beehives showed a significant reduction in bees returning to them. Bees, like birds, use the earth's natural magnetic field to navigate. Since the implementation of smart meters in my neighborhood a couple of years ago, I've noticed a significant decrease in bees in my garden and birds at the feeders, especially pigeons. Pigeons are notorious for using the earth's magnetic field to guide them. Around the world, carrier, or messenger, pigeons have earned their names because of their unique skills.

If EMFs are not to blame, are the bees dying from overexposure to herbicides and pesticides sprayed on plants? Could it also be that the combination of EMFs and environmental toxins is exponentially deadly to bees? Since I do not use chemical herbicides or pesticides, my bet is on EMFs for the cause of CCD. Of course, this could be a coincidence, and something else entirely is causing CCD. In any case, if this dire problem isn't solved in the near future, humans, along with many more thousands of species of animals, may be added to the list of endangered species.

While some individuals appear to have no problem with EMFs, others are very sensitive. A 21st-century condition called electromagnetic hypersensitivity (EHS) has emerged. A group of individuals with EHS lives in Green Bank, West Virginia, because it is in the middle of National Radio Quiet Zone, where mobile phones, radio, television transmitters, and Wi-Fi are forbidden.[6]

Previous studies of EMF exposure have found that people living near cell-tower base stations experience increased cancer risk, concentration problems, depression, dizziness, headaches, decreased libido, memory loss, skin rashes, sleep disturbances, increased suicide rates, *tremors*, and other neurological effects.[7] Other common symptoms of excessive EMFs include fatigue, heart palpitations, irritability, muscle aches, and tinnitus. Unfortunately, most people attribute these symptoms to stress, diet, or something other than EMFs. There is also strong evidence that long-term exposure to low-frequency magnetic fields is associated with lower melatonin levels. This may explain why one of the first symptoms that people notice from excessive EMFs is insomnia. Lack of sleep can cause irritability and anxiety, which can also worsen tremors.

Those with ET, and other neurological conditions, may be more sensitive to EMFs than the average population. Reducing exposure to them may help lessen the frequency and intensity of tremors, in addition to decreasing risk of brain cancer, memory loss, and sleep problems. Below are some practical recommendations.

- **Wireless electronics.** Connect or wire all wireless electronics such as computers, printers, and routers. For the computer, run an Ethernet cable from the router. For the printer, use a USB cable. Disable the wireless settings on your computer, printer, and router. If you have a Kindle or device that requires wireless Internet, you can always enable the wireless setting on your router temporarily when you need it.
- **Cordless phones.** Replace cordless phones with corded phones, especially if they are DECT phones. The base of a DECT cordless phone pulses radiation even when not in use. Older cordless models pulse radiation only when in use.
- **Mobile phone.** All mobile phones emit high levels of radiation and should be used with caution. 4G or higher smart phones are the worst offenders because they emit more radiation than the older flip-phone models. How much radiation is absorbed by the body is estimated using a measure called the specific absorption rate (SAR). Regardless of what phone you have, you should never hold an active cell phone next to any part of your body unless you don't plan to have children or don't fear cancer or dementia. Keeping the phone a few inches away from your body will decrease the amount of radiation absorbed dramatically. Better yet, keep your mobile phone off when it's not in use. Turn it on to retrieve messages and return calls a few times throughout the day. You can also use the speaker or texting feature instead of holding the phone to your ear. Do not place a turned-on mobile

phone under your pillow or next to you while you sleep. Turned-on phones send out intermittent signals to nearby cell towers even when not in use. Preferably, shut it off at night, or place it at least five feet away from your bed.

- **Video-game consoles.** The best thing to do if you have a video-game console is to sell it. If you must have one, use one that keeps you moving, such as the Nintendo Wii. Limit the time you use a video-game device, and unplug it from the electrical outlet when not in use.

- **Electronic tablets.** It is better to use a laptop that can be wired than a tablet that is wireless all the time. Like cell phones, these devices frequently send signals to wireless routers or Wi-Fi towers. Every time they do, they emit radiation. For those who like to read books on tablets, black-and-white e-readers are the safest. Just make sure that the Wi-Fi is disabled when the Internet is not being used.

- **Microwave ovens.** EMFs are strongest up to six feet from a microwave oven, so stand at least that distance from it when in use.

- **Smart meters.** Sold as energy-saving devices, these meters emit radiation, infringe on privacy, and are possible fire hazards. Some electric companies allow customers to opt out of them, usually for a fee. However, this can be futile for avoiding EMFs if your neighbors have smart meters and they are within 30 feet of your house. Still, you should opt out of the smart meter, if possible, and protest their installation and opt-out fees. The less radiation exposure your body receives, the better for your health. If you are unable to opt out, make sure your bed is not against a wall that has a smart meter on the outside of that wall. Place it as far from the smart meter as possible. The worse possible situation would be living in an apartment with a bank of smart meters for the entire apartment complex on a wall outside your apartment. In that case, your only option is to move.

- **Dimmers and CFL bulbs.** Dimmer switches and CFL bulbs emit much higher EMFs than regular, nondimmer switches and incandescent or LED bulbs. CFL bulbs also contain mercury, making cleanup of a broken bulb a dangerous affair.

- **Electronics in the bedroom.** Move electric alarm clocks and radios at least five feet from your bed. Replace products that attract EMFs including waterbeds, metal-frame beds, and electric blankets. Coil mattresses may also be a problem. A Swedish study found that mattress coils acted as antennas, drawing radiation to the bed and causing increased risk of cancer in the left breast (because most people sleep on their right sides). Maximum radio-frequency wavelength occurs about 75 cm (30 inches) above the bed coils; that is, right around the left-breast area.[8] The same correlation does not exist in Japan where people sleep on futons that are coil free. Incidence of breast cancer in Japan was equal between both breasts.

- **Get grounded.** Walking, standing, or sitting with bare feet on the ground for 15 minutes a day reduces the negative effects of EMFs. Emerging evidence shows that contact with the earth, whether barefoot outside, or indoors connected to a grounded conductive system, may be a simple, natural, and effective environmental strategy against chronic stress, autonomic nervous system dysfunction, inflammation, pain, poor sleep, and many common health disorders, including cardiovascular disease.[9]

An inexpensive way to test magnetic fields is with a small AM/FM radio set at a lower AM frequency. Static can be heard when the radio is placed close to a dimmer switch, CFL bulb, computer, or TV. A radio cannot measure the actual level of EMF radiation, but it can indicate which areas to avoid. This method does not test for wireless radio frequency (RF) from cell towers or smart meters; that requires an RF meter. EMF and RF meters can be purchased for about $100 and more. Price depends on the quality and sensitivity of the meters. See Resources for purchase information.

Many products on the market claim to shield from radiation. Unfortunately, most are expensive and have not been proven in studies. For some people, the only solution is to move to a neighborhood where cell towers, Wi-Fi towers, and electrical transformers are far from homes, and the homes are a good distance from each other. However, this is getting increasingly difficult.

NR12

Household Chemicals

*I learned a long time ago that minor surgery is when they
do the operation on someone else, not you.*

~ BILL WALTON

THERE ARE OVER 84,000 manufactured chemicals on the market and in
the environment today. Many commercial household products contain neurotoxic and carcinogenic chemicals. It should be no surprise that
neurological diseases and certain cancers are on the rise in the world.
Excessive exposure to some of these chemicals can cause or trigger
tremors. Below are the most common household products that contain tremor-inducing chemicals, followed with safer and more natural
alternatives.

Weed Killers
Weed killers are the most common herbicide used on the planet. Most
people have more exposure to herbicides than any other chemical.

Farmers spray them on millions of acres of land each year. Homeowners spray gallons of chemicals every spring and summer with the goal of achieving perfectly manicured lawns.

Research has shown that people who grow up or work on farms that use herbicides have a much higher risk of developing cancer, especially lymphomas, than those who do not. They also have a higher risk of developing neurodegenerative problems and related diseases such as dementia, Parkinson's, and ALS.[1]

America's obsession with lawns is ridiculous. The chemical runoff from lawns sprayed with herbicides ends up in groundwater. In California, 40 percent of water usage is for landscape irrigation. Grass requires significantly more water than trees. Trees provide shade, oxygen, and sometimes food. One tree, on average, produces enough oxygen in a season equivalent to what 10 people use in a year. Grass, on the other hand, just looks nice and feels good under bare feet. California is in a severe drought, but green, lush lawns are still everywhere. It's truly sad that using your property to grow food is forbidden in many areas of the United States, while it is fine to grow something you can't eat while polluting the water supply.

The chief ingredient in most herbicides all over the world is glyphosate, such as in Monsanto's Roundup. Its use is escalating along with the rising use of GM crops. Not by coincidence, the manufacturer of Roundup is also the creator of most GM seeds.

Most corn, soy, and cotton currently grown in the United States are genetically engineered to resist glyphosate. Prior to the creation of GM crops, it was not possible to spray large amounts of herbicide to kill weeds without killing the food crops too. This means that there is much more herbicide in the food we eat and the cotton clothes we wear than 30 years ago. In lab studies, Roundup and other glyphosate herbicides caused genetic damage to human and animal cells. Other studies have shown that glyphosate caused reduction of hormones and increased risks of miscarriage and attention deficit disorder.[2] Some weeds have become resistant to glyphosate, requiring farmers to use more every season. Several "superweeds" are now completely impervious to glyphosate, resulting in calls for an even stronger killer, such as 2,4-D, a chemical that has been linked with ALS, cancer, and Parkinson's.

Living near agricultural areas or golf courses is particularly dangerous. In agricultural areas, you are breathing *and* drinking the chemicals, because they eventually end up in the water supply. The grass on most golf courses is heavily sprayed with chemical herbicides, fungicides, and pesticides. How do you think they always look so nice? If you are an avid golfer or have a house on the edge of a golf course, you are probably being slowly poisoned. Some golf course managers are making an effort to reduce the chemicals they use. If the club you golf at or live by uses lawn chemicals, ask the course manager to switch to safer methods for the health of the players and the environment. If your request is denied, find out when the chemicals are sprayed, and avoid golfing or spending time outside (if you live nearby) for a couple of days afterwards. In addition, make a habit of leaving your shoes by the door when entering your house; otherwise, you'll bring the toxins into your home. Small children and pets are especially vulnerable since they spend most of their time in close proximity to the floor.

Bug Killers

Bug killers, or pesticides, were created from the nerve gases of chemical warfare. Each year, Americans use over four billion pounds of pesticides in agriculture, industry, home, and garden. Every day, Americans are unknowingly exposed to a variety of pesticides in food, drinking water, homes, schools, and offices.

Pesticides cause neurological damage to the CNS (brain and spinal cord). They inhibit the enzyme acetyl cholinesterase, which controls the metabolism of the neurotransmitter acetylcholine. Neurotransmitters are chemicals in the brain that are responsible for the health of the CNS, mood, and cognitive ability.

Pesticides are also endocrine disruptors, meaning that they impede normal functioning of the glands that produce hormones. They do this by mimicking estrogen in the body; the result is excessive stimulation or blockage of the body's natural hormones. The interrelated workings of the glands and organs that compose the endocrine system are very complex. They have been compared to the instruments in a symphony orchestra. One out-of-tune player can disrupt the harmony of the whole orchestra. This is why hormonal imbalances are linked to many health problems. They can cause or worsen ADHD, Alzheimer's, cancer, dementia, depression, dizziness, diabetes, endometriosis, fatigue, headaches, heart palpitations, hyperactivity, hypothyroidism, infertility, insomnia, memory loss, nausea, neuropathy, panic attacks, Parkinson's, tremors, and many more conditions.

In one study at the University of California, researchers found that the pesticide maneb combined with the herbicide paraquat increased the risk of developing Parkinson's disease by 75 percent.[3] The study participants were located in the Central Valley of California, where this combination of chemicals is commonly sprayed.

Permethrin and pyrethrin are other toxic pesticides commonly sprayed on alfalfa, cotton, corn, and wheat crops. They are also used in mosquito fogging and for control of mites, fleas, ticks, ants, and termites. Many flea and tick control products for dogs contain permethrin and pyrethrin. Side effects of these products in dogs include diarrhea, lack of coordination, lethargy, nausea, seizures, tremors, and vomiting. Small dogs, due to their size, and small children, who like to hug their pets, are most vulnerable to neurological damage and possibly cancer from these products. Yet, it is okay to spray these poisons over neighborhoods to kill mosquitoes in a practice called mosquito fogging.

Mosquito fogging does little to stop mosquitoes in the long term, but its chemicals kill beneficial insects, such as bees, and harm wild animals as well as humans, especially small children and pets. If mosquito fogging is scheduled for your area, you should protest it. If that fails, keep your family and pets indoors while it is going on and for at least 12 hours afterward. I would also recommend watering your lawn before letting your children and pets back outside to play on it.

Pesticides are stored in body fat. They can leak out slowly for weeks, months, or even years. Symptoms can be delayed, especially for overweight individuals. Some people become ill when losing significant weight because their bodies release these toxins. This delayed response to toxins may be one reason many people fail at dieting. It is difficult to stay on a diet if you don't feel well.

Volatile Organic Compounds

The EPA estimates that the average person spends 90 percent of his or her time indoors. Houses today are made tighter to keep heat from escaping in the winter and to keep warm air outside in the summer. This is great for lowering utility bills but not for reducing indoor air pollution. Indoor air pollution can have a worse effect on health than outdoor air pollution due to volatile organic compounds (VOCs) trapped inside the house.

VOCs are organic chemicals that have very low boiling points, so they can off-gas dangerous fumes at normal room temperature. VOCs range from mildly to highly toxic. Most scents, fragrances, and odors are made from VOCs. Those that are dangerous to human health or cause harm to the environment are regulated by law, especially for indoor use, where concentrations are the highest. Typically, most VOCs are not acutely toxic for short-term exposure; however, they can compound effects on health if exposure is long term. Some VOCs are known to cause cancer in animals, and some are suspected or known to cause cancer in humans.

Common symptoms from exposure to VOCs are allergic skin reactions, anxiety, cognitive decline, conjunctivitis, dizziness, headaches, irritation of the upper respiratory tract and eyes, kidney dysfunction, lack of coordination, mood and behavioral changes, memory loss, nausea, neuropathy, sleepiness, *tremors*, unconsciousness, visual disorders, and vomiting. Long-term exposure increases risk of damage to the liver, kidneys, immune system, and other systems and organs.

The most common organic compounds found in homes are acetone, benzene, ethylene glycol, formaldehyde, methylene chloride, perchloroethylene, toluene, xylene, and 1,3-butadiene.

Acetone is a chemical solvent used to dissolve other substances. It is found in cleaning products, nail-polish remover, and paint.

Benzene is a natural part of crude oil, gasoline, and cigarette smoke. It is also used to make certain lubricants, rubbers, dry-cleaning products, dyes, detergents, drugs, pesticides, and chemicals that produce plastics, resins, nylon, and synthetic fibers.

Ethylene glycol is used in the manufacture of polyester fibers, polyethylene terephthalate resins (PET) used in making plastic bottles, and in antifreeze. Antifreeze is very dangerous to small children and pets because they are attracted to its sweet taste; many have become seriously ill or died from ingesting it. Antifreeze should be kept in a locked cabinet or on an out-of-reach shelf.

Formaldehyde is a known carcinogen and destroyer of the CNS, yet it is in many common products. It is primarily used for making pressed-wood products such as particleboard and plywood. Particle board is used in subflooring, shelving, cabinetry, furniture and plywood is used in fencing, flooring, paneling, and roofing. Formaldehyde can also be found in glues for manufacturing automotive parts, paints, inks, synthetic carpets, vaccines, some cleaning products, and textiles for preventing colors from running and fabric from wrinkling.

Methylene chloride is predominantly used as a solvent in paint strippers and removers and as a propellant in aerosols for paints, automotive products, and insect sprays. It is also used in the manufacturing of drugs, as a fumigant for grains and strawberries after harvesting, and on citrus fruit for degreening. Workers exposed to methylene chloride have increased risk of cancer.[4]

Perchloroethylene, also known as tetrachloroethylene, is widely used in dry-cleaning fabrics and metal-degreasing operations. Studies of people exposed to it in the workplace have found associations with several types of cancers, including bladder cancer, non-Hodgkin's lymphoma, and multiple myeloma. The EPA has classified tetrachloroethylene as likely to be carcinogenic to humans.[5]

Toluene is a gasoline additive for improving octane ratings. It is also used as a solvent in paints, coatings, synthetic fragrances, adhesives, inks, cleaning products, dyes, pharmaceuticals, plastic soda bottles, nylon, cosmetic nail products, and organic chemicals. Human studies have reported developmental effects such as CNS dysfunction, attention deficits, and minor craniofacial and limb anomalies in the children of pregnant women exposed to high levels of toluene or mixed solvents.[6]

Xylenes are used as solvents, cleaning agents, and paint thinners and in the printing, rubber, and leather industries. They are also found in small amounts in airplane fuel and gasoline.

1,3-butadiene is one of the most produced chemicals. Each year, 3 billion pounds are produced in the United States, and 12 billion are produced globally. Exposure to 1,3-butadiene is an occupational hazard in industries that produce or work with agricultural fungicides, fossil fuels, petroleum refining, raw material for nylon, lead smelters, and synthetic latex and rubber. Exposure can also occur from automobile exhaust, cigarette smoke, or polluted air and water near chemical, plastic, or rubber facilities, in addition to consuming foods contaminated from plastic or rubber containers.[7] 1,3-butadiene is classified by the EPA as a known carcinogen. Several human epidemiological studies have shown an increase in cardiovascular diseases and cancer from chronic or long-term exposure to 1,3-butadiene.[8]

—ɯ—

The following recommendations can significantly reduce exposure to common household chemicals.

- **Buy green cleaning products.** Substitute commercial chemical products with those made with biodegradable ingredients. Companies that sell natural cleaning products include Seventh Generation, Green Works, and Mrs. Meyer's.
- **Make natural cleaning products.** Save a bundle by making your own cleaning products. For an all-purpose cleaner, combine one-third cup of vinegar, two-thirds cup of water, and a couple of drops of essential oil in a spray bottle and shake (with the sprayer closed). This solution cleans windows, bathrooms, and most furniture. For cleaning toilets, sprinkle some baking soda

on stains and then spray the all-purpose cleaner on the baking soda to activate it. Wait 15 minutes and scrub. Baking soda can also remove stains from synthetic carpets. Just sprinkle some on the stain and spray a little vinegar over it for extra potency. Let it dry completely and vacuum.

- **Make a natural wood polish.** Combine one part freshly squeezed lemon juice to two parts olive oil. Lemon juice can be substituted with vinegar and a few drops of lemon essential oil.

- **Paint with low- or no-VOC products.** Replace toxic paints with paints with no or low VOCs. Good brands include Benjamin Moore EcoSpec, Yolo Colorhouse, Harmony Interior Latex, and Green Planet.

- **Stop painting your nails.** Most nail polish contains formalde-hyde, toluene, dyes, and other chemicals. Acetone is the primary ingredient of nail-polish remover. Breathing it can cause irrita-tion to the respiratory tract. Nails are very porous and chemicals easily find their way into your body. Spend the money saved on healthier food and supplements or purchase non-toxic nail pol-ishes and removers. Reasonably-priced, non-toxic brands include Honeybee Gardens, Piggy Paint, Suncoat, and Zoya.

- **Wear clothes that don't need dry cleaning.** Most people spend several times more money on dry cleaning a garment than they paid for it. Purchase clothes that can be machine washed. For any garments that must be dry-cleaned, find a "green" dry cleaner that doesn't use toxic chemicals. If that is not possible, take the plastic off the clothes and air them out in the garage (or another room not used for sleeping) for a couple of days before wearing or hanging in the bedroom closet.

- **Switch to an electric lawn mower.** Gasoline fumes are very toxic. Next time your gasoline-operated lawn mower or power tool stops working, switch to an electric or battery-operated one. In the meantime, wear an N95 mask when using gasoline-oper-ated items.

- **Replace synthetic carpets.** The American Lung Association states that new carpet, as well as the adhesives and padding used during installation, can be a source of VOC emissions and act like a sponge for chemical pollutants. For example, lawn pesticides can be tracked into your home and remain in the carpet fibers. Leave shoes at the door and opt for natural flooring such as hardwood, bamboo, cork, tile, or no-emission carpeting with natural fibers such as sisal or wool. If you are unable to replace your carpet right now, vacuum it several times per week and clean it with natural products to minimize chemical exposure. Vacuum it daily if it was recently installed and still has a new-carpet smell. As long as it has that new-carpet smell, it's out-gassing toxic chemicals. Also, open the windows as much as possible to allow the chemicals to escape.

- **Remove chemicals from the bedroom.** Most mattresses contain considerable amounts of synthetic and chemical-based foams, plastics, and artificial fibers. Most box springs are made with chemically-treated wood and chemical adhesives. Consider a mattress made from natural fibers. One with no coils is even better, especially for those sensitive to EMFs. In the meantime, mattress covers made of barrier cloth can help isolate the mattress and box spring. Most bed sheets are made from GM cotton and have a formaldehyde-resin finish to make them easy care, water resistant, and shrink resistant. Never put non-organic sheets on the bed before machine washing them with a natural detergent— preferably two to three times. Sheets made from organic cotton and natural dyes are much safer, but more expensive. Since one-third of life is spent in the bedroom, this is the place to splurge and get the best quality products.

- **Buy formaldehyde-free furniture and fixtures.** Phase out particleboard furniture, cabinets, shelving, and office desks with pieces made of natural materials such as hardwood, rattan, and iron. They are more expensive but will last a lifetime compared to composite furniture and cabinets that fall apart easily and are toxic. For what can't be replaced, applying a sealant, like Safecoat, can significantly reduce the off-gassing of formaldehyde.

- **Get rid of your lawn and xeriscape.** Xeriscaping is a type of landscaping that reduces dependency on supplemental water and chemical pesticides and herbicides. Grass is replaced with landscaping that is more natural to the area. Xeriscaping is used predominately in the Southwest where rainfall is low, but it can be done anywhere. Besides saving money on the water bill and gasoline for lawn-care equipment, xeriscaping reduces the need for weed killers and the need to spend time mowing. Xeriscaping can look as, or more, appealing than a grassed landscape. For those that can't do without a lawn, a small one that is maintained properly through regular feeding, aeration, watering, and mowing should only need occasional attention to small problem areas.
- **Use natural herbicides.** If you have a small lawn or garden, the easiest way to prevent weeds is to pull them regularly before they get out of hand. Weeds can be also be prevented from germinating in lawns by applying a natural preemergent herbicide, such as corn-gluten meal, during the first warm spell in spring and in the early fall.
- **Use natural pesticides.** There are many good natural products and natural ways to get rid of pests without having to resort to toxic chemicals. Search the Internet or call your local nursery for advice.
- **Buy organic cotton.** Cotton crops are one of the heaviest sprayed. Cotton clothes expose you to doses of chemicals that can be absorbed through the skin, especially when you sweat. Organic cotton clothes are preferable but can be difficult to find. Wash non-organic cotton clothes in warm or hot water (if pre-shrunk) with detergent a couple of times before wearing.
- **Buy organic: the dirty dozen.** Stay away from eating "the dirty dozen," or the 12 most heavily sprayed crops. For 2016, they include strawberries, apples, nectarines, peaches, celery, grapes, cherries, spinach, tomatoes, sweet bell peppers, cherry tomatoes, and cucumbers. Learn to grow these crops yourself or

purchase them from a local farmer who grows them organically (but may not have USDA certification due to the cost). There is plenty of information on the Internet about organic gardening. A local nursery can be helpful too. Another option is to buy into community-supported agriculture (CSA). The CSA share gets you a subscription to a local farmer's harvest. Every week throughout the farming season, you receive (or pick up) a basket of produce. Go to www.localharvest.org to find local participating farmers.

NR13

Toxic Metals

My doctor gave me six months to live, but when I couldn't pay the bill he gave me six months more.

~Dick Wilson

METALS THAT CAN negatively affect health include aluminum, cadmium, chromium, cobalt, copper, iron, lead, manganese, nickel, and mercury. Lead is the only metal that has been linked to Tremor in several studies. However, excess levels of aluminum, copper, iron, manganese, and mercury have been associated with neuron destruction, so they are worth discussing along with lead.

Aluminum

Recent studies have shown that a small but still considerable amount of aluminum can cross the blood-brain barrier. The amount differs based on the health of a person's gastrointestinal tract. While aluminum may not be a direct cause of neurological degeneration, it is certainly involved in

Alzheimer's disease (AD).[1] People with AD have higher levels of aluminum in affected areas of their brains.

The average person ingests about seven to nine milligrams of aluminum per day. It can be found in some antacids, astringents, buffered aspirin, food additives, antiperspirants, cosmetics, vaccines, water bottles, and food products such as flour, baking powder, and anticaking and coloring agents. Excessive use of antacids, baking products with aluminum, drinking from aluminum cans and water bottles, and cooking with aluminum pots are the most common causes of aluminum toxicity.

Antacids are used for heartburn and contain 300 to 600 mg of aluminum per tablet. If you consume antacids regularly, your brain is collecting aluminum like dogs collect bones. Sometimes, antacids work only temporarily because heartburn is more often due to a lack of stomach acid rather than an excess. The stomach needs hydrochloric acid (HCl) to digest food. When HCl is low, the remaining acid in the stomach can overcompensate and cause discomfort.

A simple test to determine if you have low stomach acid is to swallow a tablespoon of apple cider vinegar following an episode of heartburn. If the heartburn dissipates, your stomach is not producing enough acid. If the heartburn gets worse, your stomach is producing too much (and, uh, sorry about that). For low stomach acid, drink some apple cider vinegar diluted in water or take a betaine HCl supplement before meals.

For excess stomach acid, stay away from foods that can trigger it. Processed foods, dairy, wheat, sugar, citrus, peppers, tomatoes, and unhealthy fats are some of the worst offenders. Natural remedies for excess stomach acid include deglycyrrhizinated licorice (DGL), aloe vera, mustard, or turmeric. My favorite is DGL. It has successfully treated gastroesophageal reflux disease (GERD) and peptic ulcers in studies. To prevent heartburn, take DGL about 20 minutes before meals (or, to relieve them, after symptoms occur).

Aloe vera keeps acid from rising by coating the esophagus. Drink a half cup of juice twice a day between meals. Aloe vera may cause diarrhea in some people when used regularly. Turmeric works by breaking down fatty foods, the cause of most acid. It can be added to food or taken as a supplement with meals. Mustard works to stop acid during an attack. Eat a half teaspoon of any gray or yellow variety.

Some medications, such as buffered pain relievers, are frequently made with aluminum. Use a nonbuffered pain reliever instead, and take it with DGL. An anti-inflammatory diet, meditation, exercise, heat or ice therapy, homeopathy, and herbs are natural ways of relieving pain. Arnica is a natural homeopathic cream used for sore muscles and injuries. Menthol sprays are also very effective.

Aluminum is frequently added to baking powder, flours, and processed foods as a preservative. Any word on the label with "alum" contained in it indicates a form of aluminum. These include sodium aluminosilicate and sodium silicoaluminate in addition to the ones that clearly include the full word "aluminum." Use only aluminum-free baking powder and flours, and avoid processed baking mixes. They contain a number of artificial ingredients in addition to aluminum. Also, stay away from drinking anything that comes in aluminum cans. Aluminum can leach into the liquid, especially with acidic drinks, such as beer and soft drinks. Someone with tremors should avoid these drinks anyway.

Aluminum is also present in most antiperspirants and some vaccines. Natural, aluminum-free deodorants are available. For a list of vaccines that contain aluminum, see NR14.

Copper

Copper is necessary for the growth, development, and maintenance of bone, connective tissue, brain, heart, and many other organs. It stimulates the immune system, supports thyroid function, helps neutralize free radicals, and maintains the strength of the myelin sheath covering the nerves. It is also required for the formation of the skin pigment melanin and for maintaining hair health and color. Copper is found in many enzymes involved in energy metabolism and is necessary for the formation of hemoglobin in the blood, along with iron. Hemoglobin is important because it helps transport oxygen throughout the body.

Copper toxicity is more common than copper deficiency because it is found in most foods, water piping, some cookware, and vitamin supplements. Copper toxicity is associated with mental and emotional disorders, behavioral problems, dizziness, headaches, vomiting, mood swings, depression, and dementia. Copper competes with zinc in the body, so excess copper decreases zinc and vice versa. Zinc is an important mineral for brain-neuron health.

There is evidence that AD has become an epidemic in developed—but not undeveloped—countries. It began in the early 1900s and has exploded in the last 50 years, leading to the conclusion that something in the environment of developed countries is a major risk factor for AD. Dr. Gregory Brewer and his team at the Southern Illinois University School of Medicine believe that the risk factor is inorganic copper leaching from plumbing. Researchers have shown that patients with AD are zinc deficient as compared to age-matched controls, which could point to excess copper decreasing the zinc. In a double-blind study led by Dr. Brewer about 20 years ago, six months of zinc therapy showed a significant cognitive benefit for mice compared to controls.[2]

Those with a rare genetic condition called Wilson's disease, affecting approximately 30,000 people worldwide, accumulate copper in the body to dangerous levels. Copper starts accumulating immediately after birth and eventually attacks the liver and brain, resulting in hepatic, psychiatric, and neurologic disorders. The symptoms, usually appearing in late adolescence, include jaundice, abdominal swelling, vomiting of blood, and abdominal pain. Tremors and difficulty walking, talking, and swallowing can occur in addition to homicidal or suicidal behavior, depression, and aggression. Women may have menstrual irregularities, infertility, or multiple miscarriages. Wilson's disease is always fatal if it is not diagnosed and treated early enough. Tests to rule it out are important if tremors started between the ages of 12 and 23.

The copper in multivitamins is inorganic and is not beneficial or necessary for health. To prevent toxicity, a multivitamin-with-minerals (MVM) supplement should have no more than two mg of copper per daily dose.

Iron

Iron is a part of all cells and, as part of hemoglobin, carries oxygen from the lungs throughout the body. Iron is also part of many enzymatic functions. Iron deficiency causes anemia, fatigue, memory loss, impaired mental abilities, and decreased immunity.

Many people are surprised to learn that too much iron in the body can be even more troubling than too little. When excess iron interacts with oxygen in the body, it produces free radicals that damage cells. Excess iron can build up in tissues and organs to cause many problems, including heart disease, liver and pancreas damage, cancer, and neurodegenerative conditions.

Early symptoms of iron toxicity include depression, fatigue, irritability, joint pain, weakness, and weight loss. More advanced symptoms are abnormal heart rhythm, shortness of breath, arthritis, loss of body hair, damage to the adrenal glands, menstruation cessation or early menopause, osteoporosis, hypothyroidism, and impotence in men.[3]

Food gives us two forms of iron. Heme iron, derived from hemoglobin, is mostly found in red meats, poultry, and fish. Nonheme iron comes from meatless sources. The best of these are legumes, tofu, seeds, broccoli, and potatoes. The body absorbs heme iron more easily then nonheme iron.

Men, children, and menopausal women do not need more iron than they get from food, so they should avoid supplements with iron. Women of childbearing age who are menstruating may need supplemental iron, especially if their diets are lacking in iron or they have heavy menstrual flows. An MVM with iron usually contains 10 to 18 mg. Those diagnosed with anemia or have symptoms of it should see their healthcare practitioners for proper dosage.

Lead

Elevated blood lead concentrations have been associated with ET in two separate studies. The first study in 2003 at Columbia University looked at the blood lead concentration of 100 ET patients and 143 controls. After adjusting for variables such as age, education, smoking, and intake of certain supplements, including vitamin C, calcium, and iron, blood lead concentrations were found to be higher in those with ET. The association was even stronger in those with no family history of ET.[4] The second study at Mersin University in Turkey measured blood lead concentrations in 105 people with ET and 105 controls. The median blood lead concentration was almost twice as high in the group with ET.[5]

Lead is extremely toxic to the body, especially for young children. Lead poisoning is less common in adults, but contamination may come from working with lead-glazed ceramics, removing lead paint, and working in the construction and plumbing fields.

The body cannot distinguish between lead and calcium, so lead is readily absorbed, especially by children and pregnant women. Symptoms of lead poisoning are numerous, including appetite loss, chronic fatigue, behavioral changes, constipation, confusion, headaches, muscle weakness, severe gastrointestinal colic, and sleep problems. Lead poisoning can lead to anemia, kidney dysfunction, memory loss, seizures, coma, and death.

Lead can turn up in drinking water, paint in old buildings, imported ceramic products, antiques, collectibles, and even garden hoses. Using a lead-free garden hose is important for watering vegetable gardens or fruit trees, because the lead from the hose ends up in the soil and then the food. Lead-free hoses usually come in white or blue colors and clearly state that they are lead-free or safe for drinking. Hoses that contain lead are particularly dangerous if they are left in the hot sun, because the heat aids the lead in leaching into the water. Always let the water run cool before using water from a warm hose, and never let children or pets drink from a hose that contains lead.

Houses in the United States built prior to 1978 are likely to contain lead paint, unless the paint has since been professionally removed. Never remove lead paint yourself. Hiring a professional is money well spent if it means saving the health of your brain.

Manganese

Manganese is an important mineral for normal brain and nerve function, bone formation, protection from free radicals, energy production, and the synthesis of L-dopamine and cholesterol. Each adult has about 15 to 20 mg of manganese stored in his or her body. Manganese deficiency and toxicity are rare; however, heavy milk and soda drinkers can become deficient because the calcium and phosphorus in these products interfere with manganese absorption.

High levels of manganese in the body usually come from drinking water, manganese supplements, or occupational exposure. High levels are associated with neurological disorders. Symptoms include appetite loss, hallucinations, headaches, leg cramps, manganism, muscle rigidity, and *tremors*. People who work as welders in steel mills and miners are at the greatest risk of manganism, a neurological disease that has symptoms similar to those of Parkinson's. People with alcoholism, liver damage, or high levels of manganese in their drinking water are also at an increased risk of neurological disorders from excess manganese.

Along with a healthy diet, the amount of manganese in an MVM is sufficient; separate manganese supplements are not beneficial unless there is a known deficiency.

Mercury

Mercury accumulates in the brain because it can cross the blood-brain barrier. It occurs in soil, water, pesticides, large fish, cosmetics, dental fillings, batteries, fluorescent light bulbs, some vaccines (see NR14), and certain medications.

Signs and symptoms of mercury toxicity include dizziness, fatigue, vomiting, hair loss, headaches, joint pain, memory problems, muscle weakness, and personality changes. Conditions that can result from too much mercury in the body include arthritis, depression, dementia, gum disease, hyperactivity, and memory loss.

Fish can contain methyl mercury, and larger fish further up the food chain accumulate more of it in their bodies. Shark, tuna, and swordfish have more mercury than salmon, shrimp, and pollock. Amalgam dental fillings contain about 50 percent mercury. Whether it can seep into the body is still a controversial subject, even among dentists. Since mercury vaporizes at high temperatures, some dentists believe that drinking hot liquids alone can release mercury from fillings. When it comes to health, it is best to err on the side of caution. Consider having amalgam fillings removed and replaced with mercury-free ones. A good holistic dentist will take caution to minimize mercury vapors during the procedure.

—∿—

Detoxing metals

Your healthcare practitioner can perform tests to measure excess levels of metals in your body. Blood tests, hair analysis, and urinalysis are common ways to detect heavy metals. Two or more therapies are usually used to remove metals from the body. Common therapies include chelation, supplements, homeopathy, diet, exercise, saunas, and massage.

Chelation is a process in which nutrients and other chelating agents such as EDTA bind with metals to remove them from the body. Chelating agents can be administered intravenously, by injection, or in certain nutritional supplements. For the IV and injection methods, go to a professional well trained in chelation. Anyone with a serious health condition, especially kidney or liver disease, should seek their doctor's approval before using these methods. EDTA is considered relatively safe, but some people have experienced headaches, nausea, vomiting, or sudden drops in blood sugar or blood pressure.

Oral chelating supplements work slower than IV and injections, but they produce fewer side effects. Supplements that chelate toxic metals from the body include vitamin C, cilantro, and chlorella (green algae). Vitamin C (5,000 mg or more daily) is effective for chelating most toxic metals. Cilantro (400 mg daily) is beneficial for chelating aluminum, lead, and mercury. Chlorella (3,000 to 5,000 mg daily) is especially helpful for chelating aluminum and mercury, but not lead. It contains the highest concentration of chlorophyll, in addition to vitamins, minerals, dietary fiber, nucleic acids, amino acids, enzymes, and growth-promoting factors. However, chlorella can make some people nauseous, especially in larger doses; it is best to start with 1,000 mg and slowly increase to the desired dose.

Many foods can also chelate metals, although not as quickly as supplements or EDTA. The best chelating foods are cruciferous vegetables (broccoli, Brussels sprouts, cauliflower, kale, mustard, and radishes), cilantro, parsley, sea vegetables (dulse, kelp, nori, and wakame), and those containing pectin (apples, beets, and carrots) or sulfur (eggs, garlic, and onions).

Last, but not least, don't forget water for flushing toxins from the body. Drink at least 6 to 10 glasses of nonfluoridated water every day. The amount of water the body requires depends on body weight, activity level, and diet. Fruits and vegetables have much higher water content than cookies and crackers. The more dry foods you consume, the more water your body requires. Fluoride is toxic to the brain and body. It weakens bones and has been shown to lower IQ in children. Drink filtered water if your tap water is fluoridated.

NR14

Vaccinations

The art of medicine consists of amusing the patient while nature cures the disease.

~VOLTAIRE

MILLIONS OF DOSES of vaccines are administered to children and adults in America each year. There is much controversy surrounding vaccinations and their safety. Many parents of autistic children swear that their children were fine before getting vaccinated. The MMR (three-in-one vaccine for measles, mumps, and rubella) and the human papilloma (HPV) vaccines are currently under attack. There have also been debates over the hepatitis B (Hep B) vaccine due to many reports of severe reactions. Studies can be misleading because the same companies that manufacture the vaccines frequently pay for the studies, a major conflict of interest. In addition, vaccines are usually tested individually and rarely in combination like they are administered. Whereas the immune system may be able to handle one or two vaccinations taken at once, several may throw it into overdrive. In a German study, researchers found that vaccinated children have two to five times more disease and disorders than unvaccinated children. The immune system pays for the prevention of diseases.[1]

In theory, vaccines are great because they help prevent many horrible diseases and their spread. Unfortunately, vaccination manufacturers add many chemicals to them that can cross the blood-brain barrier and cause damage, including aluminum, mercury, and formaldehyde.

Aside from the autism controversy, there are many less severe but troubling potential vaccine reactions. Abdominal pain, cough, diarrhea, dizziness, fatigue, fever, headaches, joint pain, muscle aches, nausea, vomiting, rash, shaking, swelling and pain at the point of injection, and swollen glands are common. More severe, but rare, reactions include brain damage, coma, deafness, fainting, high fever, pneumonia, severe allergies, and seizures.

So why do manufacturers add chemicals to vaccines? According to the CDC, ensuring that vaccines are potent, sterile, and safe requires minute amounts of chemical additives that inactivate a virus or bacteria, stabilize the vaccine, and help to preserve and prevent the vaccine from losing its potency over time. Although the amount of additives may be "minute" per vaccine, the problem with some of them, such as aluminum and thimerosal, is their ability to collect in the brain.

By 15 months of age, infants have received approximately 36 vaccines. The CDC states that the main reasons for grouping so many vaccines into fewer injections are to lessen the risk of a child getting any of the target diseases, lower costs for the parents, and reduce the trauma of getting so many separate injections. More and more parents, however, are skipping or delaying vaccines. Some are foregoing vaccines for "less risky" diseases such as the flu and chicken pox, and some parents are spreading them out over a longer time, hoping to reduce the possibility of a severe reaction.

Hepatitis B, a liver disease, can only be contracted through sexual contact or bodily fluids, yet the Hep B vaccine is given at birth. Some reactions to it include convulsions, diarrhea, excessive sleeping, fever, hives, prolonged crying, rashes, shock, vomiting, and serious changes in mental, emotional, or physical behavior.[2]

The human papilloma virus is a sexually transmitted infection that can cause cancer. The HPV vaccine is a three-dose vaccine that is recommended for girls and boys starting at 11 or 12 years of age. It does not prevent all strains of HPV, thereby giving the recipient a false sense of security. The HPV vaccine has caused some of the most severe, albeit rare, reactions, including dizziness, nausea, paralysis, vomiting, and the autoimmune disease Guillain-Barré. There have even been claims of death following injection.[3] The general public may dismiss these reactions as rare, but the parents of children who have them can't do that.

Most people do not report reactions to vaccines because their doctors usually shrug them off as something else. Even if a doctor doesn't validate it, a reaction should be reported on the Vaccine Adverse Event Reporting System (VAERS) website or by calling 1-800-822-7967. The ingredients in vaccines won't change if the FDA believes that there are few problems with them.

Discussed below are some of the most common and frequently used ingredients in vaccines.[4] For a complete list of ingredients by vaccine and brand, go to the CDC website and search "Appendix B-Pink Book."

Aluminum
Adjuvants, in the form of gels or salts of aluminum, help promote an earlier, more potent, and more persistent immune response to a vaccine. Aluminum is present in the diphtheria-pertussis (DT and Td), diphtheria-tetanus-pertussis (DTaP and Tdap), Hepatitis A (Hep A), Hepatitis B (Hep B), Haemophilus influenzae type b (PredvaxHIB brand), HPV, meningococcal (Bexsero brand for meningitis), and pneumococcal (Prevnar brand) vaccines. Aluminum is not present in most influenza vaccines, polio vaccines, or live viral vaccines such as those that prevent measles, mumps, rubella, chicken pox, shingles, and rotavirus.

Animal-derived products
Animal-derived products in vaccines include amino acids, glycerol, detergents, gelatin, enzymes, and blood. Cow milk is a source of amino acids and sugars such as galactose. Glycerol is a cow-tallow derivative. Gelatin

and some amino acids come from cow bones. The flu and yellow-fever vaccines, which are prepared using chicken eggs, contain egg protein. Ordinarily, people who can eat eggs or egg products can safely take these vaccines.

Bovine-calf serum is found in the MMR (ProQuad), polio, and shingles vaccines. The serum is produced from whole blood collected from calves up to 16 to 18 months of age and of either sex, with no breed predominance. The quarantined herds are under veterinary supervision and monitored for various bovine diseases.

Bovine albumin, or protein, is found in the Hep A, Haemophilus influenzae type b (Hib), and pneumococcal (Prevnar) vaccines. Bovine muscle tissue, extract, and/or casein are found in the DT, DTaP and Tdap vaccines. Fetal bovine serum is in the MMR (MMR-II) and Varicella (chicken pox) vaccines.

Monkey kidney is in the polio vaccines and canine kidney is in the Flucelvax brand of the flu vaccine. Porcine gelatin is in the FluMist (spray for influenza) and Zoster (shingles) vaccines.

MRC-5 and WI-38, or human diploid cells (derived from aborted fetuses), are in the Hep A, MMR, Zoster, and Varicella vaccines. Lung cells were taken from an aborted fetus in the 1960s and used to produce cells that are of a consistent genetic makeup. These cell lines are used as cultures to grow live viruses that are used in these vaccines.

Human serum albumin (protein found in blood plasma) is found in the MMR and Varicella vaccines. The form found in the MMR-II vaccine has recombinant (genetically modified) DNA. The Hep B vaccines also have recombinant DNA obtained from yeast cells.

Antibiotics

Some vaccines include antibiotics to prevent the growth of bacteria during production and storage. They are present in the Hep A, MMR, polio, Zoster, Varicella, and some of the influenza vaccines. No vaccine produced in the United States contains penicillin.

Formaldehyde
Formaldehyde inactivates bacterial products in toxoid vaccines. These vaccines use an inactive bacterial toxin to produce immunity. Formaldehyde also kills unwanted viruses and bacteria that might contaminate the vaccine during production. Most vaccines incorporate formaldehyde, including DT, Td, DTaP, Tdap, Hep A, Hep B, influenza (certain brands), meningococcal (certain brands), and polio vaccines. Formaldehyde is currently not in the HPV, MMR, and Varicella vaccines. According to the CDC, *most* formaldehyde is removed from a vaccine before it is packaged.

Monosodium glutamate (MSG)
Used as a stabilizer, MSG is found in the FluMist influenza, MMR, Zoster, and Varicella, vaccines. Stabilizers help the vaccine remain unchanged when it is exposed to heat, light, acidity, or humidity.

Thimerosal
Thimerosal is a mercury-containing preservative used in vaccines to prevent contamination with and growth of potentially harmful bacteria. Thimerosal has been removed from most vaccines but unfortunately still exists in the multidose influenza, multidose meningococcal, and Td (Decavac) vaccines.

—∞—

Aluminum, mercury, and MSG are toxic to the brain even in small amounts. Some studies show elevated aluminum levels in the brains of those who had Alzheimer's disease. Mercury has damaging consequences on the nervous system, and studies outside the United States have linked it to autism. As previously discussed, MSG is an excitotoxin that crosses the blood-brain barrier, kills neurons, and can trigger or cause symptoms of shaking. Formaldehyde is a carcinogen. Removing most of this poison, but not all, is not a comforting thought.

How many vegans or vegetarians know that the vaccine they receive may contain bovine muscle tissue, fetal bovine serum, or monkey kidney? Most vaccines contain at least one, if not several, animal products. Vegans and vegetarians have no other alternative if they want to be vaccinated.

Like the HPV vaccine, the flu vaccine only protects against specific strains of the flu. You may get a different strain of flu than the vaccine was meant to protect you from. Those with moderate-to-severe egg allergy should avoid vaccines containing egg protein. Currently, only the flu shot and yellow fever vaccines contain egg protein. The FluMist spray vaccine is an alternative for the flu shot, but it is a "live" vaccine that should be taken with caution. According to the CDC, pregnant women, those with chronic medical conditions, and those younger than 2 years or older than 49 years of age, or those younger than 20 years of age on aspirin therapy should not take FluMist.

The most common immunization given to adults is the flu vaccine. Vaccines to prevent shingles and pneumonia are also recommended by the CDC for older adults. Only you and your healthcare practitioner can decide whether getting a particular vaccine is worth the risks. If you are vaccinated, take plenty of vitamin C and chlorella before and after the injection to help detox the heavy metals, excitotoxins, or other additives.

There is another choice. If you have a strong immune system, shingles, pneumonia, and influenza are preventable. Below is a list of 10 ways to build immunity naturally. These are important habits to practice even if you decide to be vaccinated.

1. **Sleep seven to nine hours per night**
   If you read NR7, you already know how important sleep is to your health. Restful sleep stimulates production of natural killer cells which attack viruses. Getting to bed regularly between 10:00 and 11:00 p.m. also helps build melatonin reserve, a powerful antioxidant.
2. **Wash your hands frequently**
   Germs travel best by hand. Everyone touches objects touched by other people, and then they touch their faces, sometimes hundreds

of times per day, without thinking about it. Always wash your hands after using the restroom and always right before eating. How many times have you visited a fast-food restaurant, handled money, and then sat down and ate without washing your hands first? A study found that paper money has viruses, MRSA and other bacteria, feces, and even semen on it. Ugh! If that doesn't trigger your gag reflex, nothing will. (It also gives phrases like "dirty money" and "money laundering" a whole new meaning.) Also, bring your own pen to the bank and department stores instead of using one that dozens of people have touched that same day.

3. **Reduce consumption of sugar and processed foods**

   In the winter months, it is more important to reduce sugar and processed foods. Be sure to eat at least five servings or more of vegetables and one to two servings of fruit per day. Fruit is high in natural sugar, so eat it with protein—such as an apple with a tablespoon of nut butter—to prevent blood sugar swings. An easier way to get your requirement of vegetables is to make batches of vegetable soup to last three or more days. Put in carrots, turnips, onions, diced tomatoes, green beans, potatoes, legumes, and broth or seasoned tomato sauce. You can add whole grains, such as barley, brown rice, millet, or quinoa, or organic chicken for a heartier soup. Top it off with turmeric, chili powder, garlic powder, sea salt, and pepper (dried jalapeno if you're a risk taker), and you have a very tasty meal. Put the leftovers in containers and place them in the fridge. My family eats this soup several times per week all winter.

4. **Drink plenty of water or tea with lemon and honey**

   Drink at least six to eight glasses of fluoride-free water or tea to help keep hydrated and flush out toxins. Add lemon and honey to tea or warm water for an extra boost. Lemon thins mucus and honey is antibacterial.

5. **Take vitamin D, garlic, and zinc**

   Unless you live where it is sunny all year and get plenty of sun exposure, taking a vitamin D supplement is important, especially during the winter months. Health experts recommend at least one gram (1,000 mg) a day.

Garlic has anti-fungal, anti-inflammatory, and antioxidant properties. It helps prevent and treat colds, athlete's foot, acne, and cold sores. Cook some every day with your food or take a good supplement like Kyolic.

Zinc increases killer cells that combat cancer, helps the immune system release more antibodies, supports wound healing, and interferes with viruses getting full access to healthy cells. Take at least 15 mg of zinc a day.

6. **Take vitamin C**

    Take at least 500 mg of vitamin C daily. Linus Pauling believes vitamin C can prevent a cold. No studies prove his theory, but that doesn't mean he is wrong. Betty White, who is 94 years of age, takes vitamin C every morning, and claims she hasn't had a cold in 20 years. I take 500 mg every day and haven't had a cold or the flu in over 10 years.

7. **Take probiotics or eat fermented foods**

    Fermented foods such as sauerkraut and miso contain probiotics for gut health. Probiotics are the good bacteria in your intestines. They keep the bad guys down so they don't have a chance to build up. Taking a probiotic supplement is also important during and after a course of antibiotics to replace the good bacteria that the antibiotics kill. See Appendix A for more discussion on probiotics.

8. **Exercise regularly**

    Exercise not only keeps you trim and fit; it boosts your immune system, stimulates neuron growth, and reduces risk of cancer. Perform activities you enjoy to prevent boredom. See Appendix C for more discussion on exercise.

9. **Avoid crowds**

    Avoid crowds during peak flu season especially where there are lots of children. Bring antibacterial wipes to the gym and wipe down the equipment's handlebars prior to use.

10. Relax

Excessive stress can decrease immunity and make it easier to catch the flu. Keep stress in check by not overworking and living a balanced life. Meditate a few minutes every day. Life is too short. Enjoy it!

—⁓—

Note on pet vaccines

Like vaccines made for humans, pet vaccines are loaded with chemicals and additives that can affect their brains and cause serious illnesses. One of my dogs had a severe allergic reaction after being vaccinated and had to be rushed to the animal hospital. Another one of my dogs developed hemolytic anemia at 18 months of age after a series of vaccinations. It took nine days at UC Davis, three blood transfusions, many sleepless nights, and about $4,000 in medical bills to save his life. He was on immunosuppressive drugs for many months after leaving the hospital. Four veterinarians that treated him said the vaccinations were the likely trigger of his disease, and all four recommended that he never receive another vaccination—doing so would risk return of the disease and his life. He never did receive another vaccination and lived to be almost 15.

One problem with pet vaccinations is the dose. Regardless of size, all dogs receive the same vaccine dose. It's ridiculous that a 10 pound dog receives the same dose as a 120 pound dog. This is probably why small dogs have more vaccine reactions than larger ones. In a pilot study performed by Dr. Jean Dodds, half-dose parvovirus and canine distemper vaccines were found to be as effective as the full-dose vaccines in dogs that weighed 12 pounds or less.[5] One holistic veterinarian in my area offers half-dose vaccines for dogs (including puppies) that weigh up to 25 pounds. If you have a small dog, request a half-dose vaccine from your veterinarian or find a holistic veterinarian that is more open to the idea.

In addition, consider spreading your pet's vaccines over several months to mitigate the risk of a reaction. Get the most critical ones first, and don't get vaccines that are not core vaccines if they are not important for your location or situation. For instance, you can forgo the Lyme vaccine if you live in an area where the risk of Lyme disease is very low. If your veterinarian is always pushing unnecessary or frequent vaccines, find another one that is more knowledgeable in the risks.

Dr. Dodds has a canine vaccine protocol and other pet health information on her website. See Resources.

Nutritional Supplements

NR15

Antioxidants

*It's bizarre that the produce manager is more important
to my children's health than the pediatrician.*

~MERYL STREEP

FREE RADICALS MAKE it harder for the body to fight off infections. They cause damage to cells that can result in damage to organs and tissues. As we age, cells are less able to cope with stress from free radicals. Starting at age 40, we lose about 5 percent of our brain volume per decade. At age 70, other conditions may start to accelerate the deterioration. Free radicals, if left unchallenged, cause and worsen chronic diseases such as cancer, diabetes, and heart disease, and neurological disorders like AD, PD, ALS, MS, and ET. Antioxidants can counter the damaging effects of free radicals and provide protection from cognitive decline, eye problems, heart disease, immune system dysfunction, and mood disorders.

Antioxidants are found primarily in fruits and vegetables. The best antioxidant-rich foods are apples, avocados, berries, cherries, asparagus, beans (red, kidney, and pinto), broccoli, garlic, leafy greens, radishes, red cabbage, sweet potatoes, and nuts. Consuming eight or more servings of organic fruits and vegetables is needed for optimum health—about three cups of vegetables and one cup of fruit a day. Unfortunately, the average American consumes an average of only two servings of vegetables (one cup) and one serving of fruit (half a cup) a day.

Consuming eight servings of fruits and vegetables is fine for preventing disease but what about those who already have a chronic condition like ET? Eight servings may not be enough. Many people struggle to consume the minimum USDA requirement of two servings of fruit and three servings of vegetables a day. This is why some people juice their produce when they are trying to heal from a chronic condition. Juicing is great, but for many, taking antioxidant supplements is more affordable and easier. Besides, juicing eliminates the fiber. A high-fiber intake is associated with lower risk of colon cancer, heart disease, obesity, and type 2 diabetes.

Neuroprotective antioxidant supplements aimed at improving brain health can be helpful in lessening or slowing the progression of ET. Think of supplementation as a preventative measure to stop free radicals in their paths before they harm healthy brain cells. The most powerful antioxidants that protect neurons are alpha-lipoic acid, astaxanthin, coenzyme Q10, curcumin, glutathione, and vitamins A, C, and E.

Alpha-lipoic acid (ALA)

ALA, also called lipoic acid, is an antioxidant that the body makes. It occurs in every cell. While some antioxidants work only in water, such as vitamin C, or in fatty tissues, such as vitamin E, alpha-lipoic acid is both fat- and water-soluble, so it works in every cell in the body. Evidence suggests that ALA may help regenerate antioxidants, making them active again after they are used up in attacking free radicals.

In several studies, ALA appears to have helped lower blood sugar levels by turning glucose into energy. The ability of ALA to kill free radicals may help people with diabetic peripheral neuropathy, which is nerve damage that causes pain, burning, itching, tingling, and numbness in the arms and legs.[1] Since ALA can reach all parts of a nerve cell, it can potentially protect nerve cells against such damage. Because ALA helps lower blood sugar, it should not be taken with diabetic drugs that do the same without monitoring by a healthcare practitioner. The combination raises the risk of hypoglycemia.

In other, separate studies, ALA reduced oxidative stress in spinal-cord injury, slowed the progression of dementia dramatically, increased glutathione and vitamin C, and improved immune T-cell function in HIV-infected patients. In animal studies, ALA also reduced the toxic effects of the anticancer drug cyclophosphamide, the immunosuppressant drug cyclosporine, and the pain pill acetaminophen.[2]

In most studies that found benefits of supplementing with ALA, several weeks of treatment were often necessary for effects to develop. There is no established dosage of ALA for Tremor; however, a dose of 30 to 100 mg per day is often recommended for optimal health. Although side effects are rare, a healthcare practitioner should monitor those who take higher amounts.

Astaxanthin

Astaxanthin comes from a microalgae called Haematococcus. The combination of its high-potency antioxidant and anti-inflammatory properties allows astaxanthin to address a vast array of health concerns. Astaxanthin acts on at least five different inflammation pathways. Most antioxidants can only handle one free radical at a time, but astaxanthin handles several simultaneously.

Studies have shown that astaxanthin is effective in protecting neurons, improving blood flow and cholesterol levels, decreasing blood pressure, boosting immunity, and preventing cataracts and macular degeneration. In one study, astaxanthin reduced oxidative damage and inflammation and enhanced immune response in young, healthy females.[3]

Another benefit of astaxanthin is its ability to work as a natural "internal" sunscreen by reducing damage caused by ultraviolet radiation from the sun. It gives the skin a healthy, tanlike "glow" as opposed to the orange coloration obtained from consuming too much beta-carotene.

Four to six ounces of wild-caught salmon provides about two to three mg of astaxanthin. Synthetic astaxanthin, produced from petrochemicals, is fed to farm-raised salmon and is not approved for human consumption in food or supplements.

There is no recommended daily allowance (RDA) of astaxanthin. Doses of supplements on the market range from 2 to 12 mg. Astaxanthin has been found to be safe at high levels. It is a fat-soluble supplement, so taking it with a small amount of fat, or food with fat in it, improves absorption.

Coenzyme Q10 (CoQ10)

CoQ10 is a powerful antioxidant that is in every cell in the body. It plays a critical role in energy production by helping convert food into energy. CoQ10 is low in most Americans and decreases with age. Certain antidepressants, diabetic drugs, diuretics, beta-blockers, and statins deplete CoQ10. Statins are particularly devastating in their ability to deplete it. The heart is usually the first organ to feel the effects due to its high energy requirement. Not replacing CoQ10 may actually increase risk of heart disease and congestive heart failure, the opposite of what statins are meant to achieve.

CoQ10 has been used and recommended for the treatment of Alzheimer's, asthma, cancer, chronic fatigue syndrome, gum disease, heart disease, and high blood pressure. Some researchers believe that CoQ10 may help with the prevention of a first heart attack or subsequent ones, because it can improve energy production in cells, prevent blood-clot formation, and act as an antioxidant.[4]

Other researchers believe that CoQ10 supplements may slow, but not cure, Alzheimer's disease. In a 2011 study, CoQ10 treatment of mice resulted in a reduction of amyloid plaque (the marker of Alzheimer's disease) and improved cognitive performance.[5] CoQ10 is still in trials for other neurodegenerative diseases such as Huntington's and Parkinson's. Preliminary evidence also suggests that CoQ10 may prevent migraines and improve immune function in those with HIV or AIDS.

Primary dietary sources of CoQ10 include oily fish such as salmon and tuna, organ meats, and whole grains. But for most people over the age of 50, dietary sources are not adequate. As a supplement, CoQ10 comes in softgels (reduced form referred to as ubiquinol) and capsules (oxidized form referred to as ubiquinone). Many manufacturers of ubiquinol claim that it is more effectively absorbed than ubiquinone based on their own studies. The only independent study I found was a small one performed by Dr. Stephen Sinatra, a cardiologist, using his own patients. His findings showed only slightly higher levels of CoQ10 in most of the patients that were taking ubiquinol, but not enough to pay the higher cost. In addition, one of his patients felt fatigue after taking *ubiquinol*, while some felt more energy after taking *ubiquinone*.[6] Furthermore, several studies have been performed using both forms of CoQ10 with positive results. So, unless you prefer the gel form or believe it is better absorbed, ubiquinone should work fine, and it costs much less.

Everyone over the age of 40 should take CoQ10 regardless of health. The recommended dosage for those in good health (few symptoms) is 30 to 50 mg daily. Those with gum disease or HBP should take 50 to 100 mg, twice daily. Those with congestive heart failure, heart disease, chronic fatigue, fibromyalgia, or who are taking statins (or have statin damage) should take 100 to 150 mg, twice daily.

Curcumin

Curcumin has anticancer, antimicrobial, antioxidant, and anti-inflammatory properties. Research has shown that curcumin is a powerful nervous system protector. The spices curry and turmeric contain curcumin. Because it can cross the blood-brain barrier, curcumin may protect against Alzheimer's and other neurological diseases. In one study, people who consumed curry with turmeric had significantly better scores on cognitive tests than those who rarely consumed it.[7] In a 2007 study, curcumin protected laboratory animals from a type of brain injury that often follows strokes.[8] In yet another study, curcumin decreased oxidative stress and improved memory in aged female rats.[9]

Curry and turmeric can be used on eggs and meats and mixed into grains and soups. Curcumin also comes in capsule form as a supplement. Look for supplements that contain 300 to 500 mg, standardized to 95 percent curcumin. Turmeric supplementation should be avoided by those with gallstones. Turmeric helps prevent gallstones by promoting gallbladder emptying, but for those with existing gallstones, it could increase the risk of symptoms.

Glutathione (GSH)

Glutathione has been called the "master antioxidant" because it keeps all other antioxidants performing at top levels. GSH is a combination of three amino acids—cysteine, glycine, and glutamine. GSH removes toxins from cells and protects the body from their damaging effects. The body produces its own GSH, but toxins from infections, medications, poor diet, pollution, radiation, and stress can deplete it, leaving the body susceptible to cell death from oxidative stress and free radicals.

According to research, GSH helps prevent aging, neurodegeneration, and diseases such as cancer, cystic fibrosis, and HIV.[10] The secret of GSH may be the sulfur it contains, one of the most important compounds in the body. Sulfur is a sticky and smelly molecule that attaches to all the bad things in the body, including free radicals and heavy metals, and removes them. GSH is critical for proper liver and immune function. The body recycles GSH except when the toxic load becomes too great. Insufficient amounts can prevent the liver from doing its job of detoxification, which can burden and damage it.

Studies have shown that GSH supplements do not raise the level of GSH in the blood, because the body digests proteins. In animal studies, only very small amounts were able to enter the bloodstream, and the effect only lasted about three hours. In addition, in mice that were chemically depleted of GSH, it rose in all organs except the liver, where it is needed most for detoxification.[11, 12] The good news is that there are several natural ways to increase the body's store of this critical molecule.

1. **Consume more sulfur-rich foods**

   Garlic, onions, leeks, chives, and the cruciferous vegetables, including broccoli, Brussels sprouts, cabbage, cauliflower, collards, kale, radishes, turnips, and watercress, are all rich in sulfur.

2. **Take GSH-supporting supplements**

   Vitamins C and E, ALA, selenium, garlic, curcumin, and silymarin (milk thistle) can help boost the body's production of GSH. Vitamins C and E work together with selenium to help the body recycle and produce more GSH. As mentioned earlier, garlic can boost GSH in the body because it contains sulfur. It also has antifungal, antiviral, and anti-inflammatory properties. Unless you consume raw garlic daily, this is a great supplement to take, especially in the winter to prevent illness. Besides raising levels of GSH, milk thistle is an herb that has long been used in the prevention of gallstones and detoxification of the liver.

3. **Take bioactive whey protein**

   Whey protein is a by-product of cheese production. It is a great source of the amino-acid building blocks for GSH synthesis. Make sure the whey protein is bioactive and made from nondenatured proteins. Denaturing refers to the breakdown of the normal protein structure.

4. **Exercise**

   Exercise increases GSH levels in addition to boosting the immune system, improving detoxification, and stimulating neuron growth.

Vitamin A

The main functions of vitamin A are to protect against night blindness, aid in the formation and growth of bones and teeth, enhance and support the immune system, and protect against colds, influenza, cancer, and heart disease. Vitamin A also helps with skin disorders such as acne, wrinkling, and age spots.

Food sources of vitamin A include apricots, asparagus, beet greens, broccoli, Brussels sprouts, cantaloupe, carrots, cherries, collards, dandelion greens, dulse, kale, lettuce, mango, mustard greens, papayas, parsley, peaches, pumpkin, red cabbage, red peppers, spinach, spirulina, sweet potatoes, Swiss chard, turnip greens, watercress, watermelon, and yellow squash.

Taking large amounts of synthetic vitamin A over long periods can be toxic, especially to the liver. Vitamin A in the form of beta-carotene does not cause problems in large amounts unless a rare condition exists in which the liver is unable to convert beta-carotene to vitamin A. The recommended daily amount of vitamin A in the form of beta-carotene is 5,000 to 10,000 IU. It is easiest to take vitamin A in a quality MVM.

Drugs that interfere with absorption of vitamin A are alcohol, antibiotics, laxatives, and some cholesterol-lowering drugs. Those who are pregnant or have liver disease should not take more than 10,000 IU per day without a doctor's approval.

Vitamin C

Vitamin C is a water-soluble nutrient that has antibacterial, anti-inflammatory, antioxidant, and antiviral properties. The main benefits of vitamin C are boosting the immune system and protecting against cardiovascular disease, prenatal health problems, eye disease, and cancer. Although vitamin C is not proven to prevent colds, it does reduce their duration. Vitamin C also enhances the benefits of exercise and helps reduce damage from smoking.

Foods that are especially rich in vitamin C are bell peppers, broccoli, Brussels sprouts, cantaloupe, cauliflower, grapefruit, kale, lemon juice, mustard greens, oranges, papaya, parsley, strawberries, and tomatoes.

Vitamin C supplements should be taken with bioflavonoids. Bioflavonoids, when combined with vitamin C, help increase collagen and protect vitamin C from oxidation. Collagen is the connective tissue found in skin, cartilage, ligaments, vertebral disks, joint linings, capillary walls, bones, and teeth. Collagen gives support and shape to the body, maintains healthy blood vessels, and helps heal wounds. It also helps prevent skin wrinkling, varicose veins, and hemorrhoids. Bioflavonoids, along with vitamin C, also reduce the amount of histamine that cells release, making them a great natural remedy for allergies and asthma.

The US recommended daily allowance (RDA) for vitamin C is 75 mg for females and 90 mg for males. The recommended dosage of vitamin C for optimal health is 500 mg per day. Vitamin C absorbs quickly in the body, so it is best to take smaller doses throughout the day when taking more than 500 mg, especially during illnesses. Vitamin C is not toxic at any level, but it can cause diarrhea at high levels. Cutting back the dosage usually fixes the problem. Kidney stones are another worry, but studies are weak in this area and stones are rare. Taking a buffered vitamin C, which contains magnesium, or a separate magnesium supplement, will prevent kidney stones. The ascorbic-acid form of vitamin C frequently comes from GMO corn, so make sure the label states that the product is GMO free or USDA organic.

Vitamin E

Vitamin E is a fat-soluble nutrient that protects the tissues of the breasts, skin, eyes, liver, lungs, and testes. It also helps protect against cardiovascular disease and cancer. The antioxidant function of vitamin E is enhanced by beta-carotene, vitamin C, flavonoids, CoQ10, and the mineral selenium. Antiaging is another benefit of vitamin E, smoothing lines and wrinkles and treating age-related brown spots.

The primary sources of vitamin E are the oil components of seeds, nuts, and grains. Vitamin E is also in cold-pressed olive oil, wheat germ oil, tofu, and spinach.

The RDA of vitamin E for adults ranges from 15 to 19 IU. For optimal health, 50 to 200 IU is recommended. The natural form of vitamin E, d-alpha tocopherol, is the most potent. Avoid dl-alpha tocopherol, the synthetic form.

Vitamin E naturally thins the blood. It should not be taken with medications that do the same. Vitamin E should also be stopped at least a couple of weeks before a surgery to reduce risk of bleeding.

NR16

B-Complex Vitamins

The best doctor gives the least medicine.

~Benjamin Franklin

B VITAMINS ARE VITAL to the health of the central nervous system, skin, eyes, hair, liver, mouth, brain, and the muscle tone of the gastrointestinal tract. They act as catalysts by accelerating biochemical reactions in the body to sustain life.

Common signs of B-vitamin deficiency are numerous and include, but are not limited to, acne, anemia, arthritis, beriberi (thiamine deficiency), blood-sugar changes, bone loss, constipation, dementia, depression, dizziness, drowsiness, edema, fatigue, forgetfulness, gastrointestinal problems, gum inflammation, graying hair, hair loss (biotin deficiency), headaches, insomnia, irritability, loss of appetite, low blood sugar, memory problems, muscle weakness, nausea, nervousness, neurological damage, pellagra (pantothenic-acid deficiency), ringing in the ears, tingling in hands and feet, and *tremors*.

There are eight B vitamins including thiamine (B1), riboflavin (B2), niacin (B3), pantothenic acid (B5), pyridoxine (B6), biotin (B7), folate or folic acid (B9), and methylcobalamin (B12). B vitamins are usually referred to with names, except B6 and B12. When combined in a dietary supplement, they are referred to as B complex.

PABA (para-aminobenzoic acid), choline, and inositol are three more components of a B-complex supplement. PABA is an antioxidant and a component of folic acid. Choline, an essential nutrient, is included in a B-complex supplement because it enhances the metabolism of folate and vitamin B12. It is sometimes referred to as the "unofficial" B vitamin because it is similar in function. Choline is critical for brain function and tremor reduction. Inositol works to enhance the benefits of choline, so they are frequently paired in supplements. Inositol is not an essential nutrient, because the body produces it. CDP-choline has been used in clinical trials for ET, Parkinson's, and cognitive impairment with promising results. There's more discussion on CDP-choline in the next chapter.

Vitamin B12 aids in the formation of red blood cells and healthy nerve tissue and works with folate, or folic acid, in the synthesis of DNA. It is also important for maintaining the health of the myelin sheath that surrounds nerve cells. Loss of myelin is the hallmark of some neurodegenerative diseases, including multiple sclerosis. Besides vitamin B12, cholesterol is a necessary nutrient for myelin, which is another good reason to stay away from cholesterol-lowering drugs. Vitamin B12 deficiency is common among the elderly due to stomach problems and other conditions that limit its absorption. People most prone to vitamin B12 deficiency are vegans, alcoholics, and people who suffer from fibromyalgia. These groups are also at higher risk of developing tremors.

Some people diagnosed with Alzheimer's or dementia may actually have a B12 deficiency or serum levels of B12 at the lower end of normal.[1] If you are at least age 50, have memory problems, tremors, or have lived a vegan lifestyle for more than a few years, you should get a baseline blood test for vitamin B12. If your test comes back at the lower end of normal, ask your doctor for vitamin B12 injections until you are at the higher end of normal. Nasal sprays are also available if injections make you queasy.

Bring a copy of the study mentioned above to show your doctor. If your doctor refuses, find another one, or go to an alternative healthcare practitioner. Saving your memory is more important than what your doctor thinks.

Although riboflavin deficiency has not been linked to tremors in studies, it looks promising for improving them, according to a pilot study at a Brooklyn, New York, medical center. Sixteen patients aged 50 to 90, 4 with head tremor and 12 with hand tremor, were given 400 mg daily of riboflavin. They were then evaluated at four-week intervals. The dose was increased to 600 mg at four weeks and then to 800 mg at eight weeks for those showing no improvement. Riboflavin decreased tremor severity in 10 patients, and in more than half of the participants, riboflavin was associated with an enhanced ability to write, eat, drink, and pour liquids. Researchers observed no adverse effects but caution that riboflavin is poorly absorbed when taken with certain medications. In addition, high doses could cause some forms of eye disease or skin sensitivities to light in certain individuals.[2] If you consider taking very high doses of riboflavin for the tremor-reducing effect, it is best to see a healthcare practitioner for dosage and monitoring.

The richest food sources of B vitamins include brewer's yeast, broccoli, carrots, cheese, egg yolks, fish, legumes, peanuts, poultry, red meat, spinach, sunflower seeds, wheat germ, whole grains, and yogurt. Other lesser sources include asparagus, avocados, bananas, beans, Brussels sprouts, kelp, leafy green vegetables, mushrooms, molasses, nuts, plums, potatoes, prunes, raisins, soybeans, spirulina, and watercress. Stay away from processed foods fortified with B vitamins like white-flour products. Any version of frankenwheat does not have the same health benefits as products made from whole-grain, low-gluten flours.

Always take B vitamins as a balanced B-complex supplement because they work in synergy. A deficiency in one usually indicates a deficiency in another. A balanced B-50 complex has 50 mg each of the B vitamins except B12, folate, and biotin. There should be at least 50 mcg each of B12 and biotin and at least 400 mcg of folate. PABA, choline, and inositol are included in B-complex supplements at varying amounts.

Is there a difference between folic acid and folate? Folic acid is the synthetic version of vitamin B9 found in most supplements, whereas folate refers to the form that occurs naturally in food. Many health professionals believe they are essentially the same but recent animal studies indicate an increased risk of cancer when taking high levels of folic acid. No human studies have been performed and the amounts used in animal studies were several times higher than the amounts found in must multivitamins. More research is needed. In the meantime, don't throw out your supplements unless you are pregnant or taking very high levels of folic acid. Many supplements now include the folate form of vitamin B9, so the next time you purchase multivitamins or a B complex, consider ones with folate. The best form is called 5-methyltretrahydrofolate (5-methyl-THF, or 5-MTHF).

For optimum health, a balance B-25 complex (or higher) is recommended. A good-quality MVM will contain at least that amount. If your MVM doesn't, you can take a separate B complex. B vitamins are water soluble, making toxic effects at high doses rare, because the excess ends up in your urine. Don't be alarmed if your urine turns bright yellow by the way. This is due to the riboflavin.

NR17

Choline

Never go to a doctor whose office plants have died.

~ERMA BOMBECK

C HOLINE IS CLASSIFIED as a B vitamin, but it is actually closer to a fat. Choline is a component of phosphatidylcholine (PC), a critical phospholipid found in cells. PC is also known as lecithin. Lecithin is important in the emulsification of fats and cholesterol in the body. Phospholipids help brain cells communicate by supporting the function of cell receptors, which serve as gatekeepers to transmit signals between the outside and inside of nerve cells. Nerve cells contain glutamate receptors that cover the cell membrane. When glutamate binds to the receptor on the outside, the receptor changes shape and opens within milliseconds, allowing ions (charged particles) to enter the cell. The process is vital for communication between nerve cells and plays a role in brain development, learning, and memory. Problems with glutamate-receptor function appear to be involved in many disorders, including autism, some types of cancer, depression, Parkinson's disease, and schizophrenia.[1]

Choline is also part of acetylcholine, one of the most abundant neurotransmitters in the body. Acetylcholine is critical for the structural integrity of the nervous system and cell membranes. It transmits signals between nerve cells and skeletal muscles. Acetylcholine is also critical for learning and turning short-term memories into long-term memories. Chronic deficiencies are associated with many neurological disorders.

A mild deficiency in choline is very common. Less than 10 percent of Americans get the recommended amount in their diet. Signs of a choline deficiency include anxiety, craving fatty foods, fatigue, insomnia, irritability, memory problems, mood disorders, and poor muscle tone.

Until recently, it was thought that the body could substitute other substances for choline, such as folate, vitamins B6 and B12, and the amino acid methionine. However, recent evidence has shown that some people cannot maintain adequate choline supplies using other nutrients and must obtain them independently through diet or choline supplements.[2] Good food sources of choline are Brussels sprouts, cauliflower, chicken, codfish, eggs, milk, and spinach.

A powerful form of choline called citicoline (cytidine 5'-diphosphocholine), or CDP-choline, became available in the late 1990s as a supplement. Citicoline is a more powerful form of choline because it contains cytidine, a component of RNA. Cytidine has been found to control glutamate levels in the brain. As discussed in NR2, high glutamate levels can speed up cell damage in the brain by exciting cells to death.

Citicoline was first approved for use in PD and stroke, but it now being used to treat Alzheimer's, glaucoma, and ET. According to a 2009 study, it was effective in the control of tremors in a study of 18 patients, comprising 8 males and 10 females, at the neurology department at King Hussein Medical Center in Jordan. A daily dose of 400 mg of citicoline presented overall improvement in 89 percent of the study group, which is higher than in any previous study on controlling Tremor. Compare these results to propranolol, an FDA-approved medication for ET, which has an average effectiveness of 50 to 60 percent in reducing tremors.[3]

An optimal dosage of citicoline, or CDP-choline, is 250 to 400 mg per day. Choline supplements are less expensive and can substitute for CDP-choline. However, keep in mind that the study referred to previously used citicoline, not choline, so although choline may help with tremors, citicoline may be more effective. It is best to take a choline supplement with a B complex for better absorption. For an additional choline boost, lecithin granules can be added to cereals, yogurts, and baking recipes. Lecithin is frequently sourced from soy products, which means it has a 90 percent chance of being genetically modified. Instead, buy USDA-organic lecithin granules, or look for "non-GMO" on the label.

NR18

Magnesium

If I knew I was going to live this long, I'd have taken bet-
ter care of myself.

~MICKEY MANTLE

MAGNESIUM IS INVOLVED in over 300 biochemical processes in the body. Some of the many critical functions of magnesium include cell growth and reproduction, DNA and RNA synthesis, blood pressure regulation, blood flow, normal heart rhythm, formation of bones and teeth, immune system support, blood glucose regulation, energy metabolism, glutathione synthesis, proper bowel elimination, muscle contractions, and proper nerve signaling. Magnesium also helps protect against cardiovascular disease and damage from environmental chemicals, heavy metals, and toxins by aiding in the detoxification process.

Magnesium is necessary for active transport of calcium and potassium ions across cell membranes, a process important for nerve signals, muscle contractions, and normal heart rhythm. A deficiency of magnesium causes diminished energy and compromises muscle and nerve functions.[1]

It has been linked to many conditions including, but not limited to, asthma, circulatory disturbances, cluster headaches, cognitive decline, dependent disorder, depression, diabetes, epilepsy, ET, fibromyalgia, heart arrhythmia, heart disease, high blood pressure, insomnia, kidney stones, migraines, muscular dysfunction, osteoporosis, Parkinson's, preeclampsia, tinnitus, and TMJ. Signs and symptoms of insufficient magnesium levels include abdominal pain, anxiety, confusion, constipation, dizziness, headaches, low blood sugar, sleeping problems, muscular spasms and weakness, sadness, tics and twitches, tight muscles, and *tremors*.

Eighty percent of people in the United States have a magnesium deficiency. The soil in which we grow our food has deteriorated considerably due to the popularity of intensive, single-crop agricultural methods, heavy use of herbicides, and agricultural practices designed to improve produce size, growth rate, and pest resistance. Donald Davis and his team of researchers at the University of Texas studied the United States Department of Agriculture's nutritional data from both 1950 and 1999 for 43 different vegetables and fruits. They found declines in the amount of protein, calcium, phosphorus, iron, riboflavin (vitamin B2), and vitamin C in the fruits and vegetables over the past half century.[2]

The problem is further complicated by the current Western diet, which contains high amounts of phosphorus from fast foods, especially processed meats and soft drinks. Phosphorus binds with magnesium, preventing its absorption. To make matters even worse, the modern Western diet contains low levels of magnesium-rich foods. When was the last time you had figs, kelp, spinach, Swiss chard, kale, avocados, bananas, nuts, pumpkin seeds, or whole grains like buckwheat, millet, and quinoa? These foods are rich in magnesium. If you're like most people, you probably had a banana or two in the past week but not any of the other foods.

A magnesium deficiency can occur for a variety of reasons other than diet and soil conditions. According to the National Institutes of Health, other causes can include alcoholism, certain medications, and a loss of fluid due to excessive urination, sweating, or diarrhea. Magnesium deficiency can also occur because of celiac disease and IBS due to malabsorption.

At the turn of the 19th century, most families had gardens. They consumed their produce hours after harvesting instead of weeks, giving them the full benefit of the food's nutrients. Today, few people have gardens. California grows most of the country's produce, which can travel hundreds to thousands of miles before it gets to the supermarket. Days later, it is sold as "fresh." It is then stored in refrigerators to keep it "fresh" even longer. Every day that fruits and vegetables go uneaten means more nutrients lost, especially for fast-decaying ones like leafy greens. Ironically, frozen produce contains higher amounts of nutrients than most "fresh" produce because they are picked at their peak ripeness, a time when they are nutrient dense, and processed immediately. The freezing process involves blanching the vegetables in hot water to kill any bacteria and to slow down enzymatic action. Then the vegetables are quickly frozen, locking in nutrients.

Magnesium is one of the most important supplements for reducing tremors. Following the advice in the *Food Choices* section will increase magnesium-rich foods in your diet. However, a magnesium supplement is still highly recommended for anyone with ET or other tremor types. This one mineral can help prevent many chronic conditions and alleviate many symptoms: anxiety, constipation, diabetes, heart disease, high blood pressure, insomnia, migraines, muscle weakness, weak bones, TMJ, and *tremors*. Magnesium helps regulate heart rhythm, so it should not be taken with drugs that do the same, such as beta-blockers or CCBs, without a doctor's approval and monitoring.

Magnesium supplements come in many forms, quality, and levels of absorption. The best forms are described here. Choose the one that best fits your needs and budget.

1. **Magnesium glycinate**
    Chelated form of magnesium with one of the highest levels of absorption. Ideal for those trying to correct a known deficiency.

2. **Magnesium taurate**

   Combination of magnesium and taurine, an amino acid that has calming effects. Magnesium taurate absorbs well and does not cause a laxative effect.

3. **Magnesium malate**

   Combination of magnesium and malic acid, a weak organic acid in apples and other fruits and vegetables. The weak bond makes it easily absorbable.

4. **Magnesium orotate**

   Easily absorbable chelated form of magnesium. Dr. Hans Nieper, a German physician, introduced it to treat and prevent heart attacks, atherosclerosis, blood clots, kidney failure, and viral disease. Magnesium orotate has also been used to treat ADHD, autism, recovery from heart attacks, coronary heart disease (in combination with potassium orotate), in addition to improving the elasticity of blood vessels and athletic performance.[3]

5. **Magnesium citrate**

   Magnesium with citric acid that causes a mild laxative effect. Has a lower concentration of magnesium but is highly absorbed (90 percent). It is one of the best forms for the price.

6. **Magnesium chloride**

   Versatile form available in capsules, powder, oil, and IV. Some researchers believe it is the best absorbed because magnesium chloride has enough extra chloride to produce hydrochloric acid in the stomach to enhance absorption.

7. **Magnesium L-threonate (MgT)**

   Dr. Liu and colleagues at Tsinghua University in Beijing, China, developed this new magnesium compound with superior ability to penetrate the mitochondrial membrane of a cell. MgT has enhanced learning in both young and aged rats. Cellular changes associated with memory revealed an increase in the number of functional synapses, activation of key signaling molecules, and an improvement of synaptic processes crucial for learning and memory.[4] MgT is expensive and has no proven advantages over other magnesium supplements, but it might be worth a try if the others aren't very effective for tremors.

Carbonate, oxide, and sulfate forms of magnesium are not recommended as daily supplements. They have more laxative effects than others and do not absorb well.

Many MVM supplements include carbonate forms of both calcium and magnesium due to their low cost. Magnesium and calcium carbonate are made from limestone and chalk and have antacid properties. If you take these supplements for their antacid properties, I would advice trying DGL instead or adding a better absorbed form of magnesium.

Magnesium oxide is found in many MVM and magnesium supplements. Magnesium hydroxide is the laxative form found in milk of magnesia, which should not be used as a supplement because it contains artificial dyes and flavors. Both can have laxative effects if taken in amounts needed for Tremor.

The sulfate form of magnesium in Epsom salt is great for bathing and relaxing tired muscles and as an occasional laxative. Taking it daily can cause gastrointestinal problems. Plus it tastes very bitter.

Glutamate and aspartate forms of magnesium should never be taken as supplements. They contain neuron-destroying properties.

The RDA for magnesium is 400 mg for men and 300 mg for women. To treat symptoms of tremors or a magnesium deficiency, take 600 mg to 1,200 mg per day. The body cannot absorb more than 600 mg at a time, so split higher doses between morning and evening.

NR19

Neurotransmitters

I'm trying to read a book on how to relax, but I keep falling asleep.

~JIM LOY

NEUROTRANSMITTERS ARE CHEMICALS that transmit signals across a synapse from one neuron to another. Many neurotransmitters are easily synthesized from amino acids, or proteins. There are more than 100 different neurotransmitters in the brain. Some neurotransmitters cause excitatory emotional responses, while others cause inhibitory responses. Neurotransmitters also carry pain sensations and cause voluntary muscle movements.[1]

Because neurotransmitters are made of protein, low-protein diets can cause amino acid deficiencies. Some disorders associated with amino acid imbalances are ADHD, confusion, chronic fatigue, depression, degenerative diseases, headaches, inflammatory disorders, insomnia, muscular diseases, neurological disorders, osteoporosis, and weak immunity.[2]

Neurotransmitters that inhibit, or calm, the nervous system are critical for reducing tremors. These include GABA (gamma-aminobutyric acid), glutamine, glycine, and theanine.

Low levels of GABA have been linked to ET. Scientists at the Université Laval in Canada noticed a decrease in GABA receptor concentrations in the cerebellum—the part of the brain that controls movement—of patients with ET.[3] GABA is found throughout the central nervous system and is the most widely distributed neurotransmitter in the brain, with 40 to 50 percent of the brain synapses containing it. GABA calms, both mentally and physically, by inhibiting brain cells from firing when a person is stressed or anxious. Prolonged stress may exhaust available GABA, increasing vulnerability to panic attacks, breathing difficulties, constant fear, headaches, diarrhea, and trembling.[4]

Glutamine is found in the nerves of the hippocampus and in many other areas of the brain. With the help of magnesium, the brain converts glutamine to GABA, which is another reason to take magnesium supplements.

Glycine decreases cravings for sugar and removes heavy metals from the body. When combined with GABA and glutamine, it slows down anxiety-related messages.

Theanine is found in green tea. Theanine converts to GABA in the brain. It also aids in the release of serotonin and dopamine. Serotonin decreases pain, boosts mood, and promotes relaxation and sleepiness. Dopamine regulates pleasure and mood, behavior, and cognition control. Significant loss of dopamine-secreting cells is the main cause of body stiffness and trembling in Parkinson's.

Levels of GABA can be increased through diet, yoga, and supplements. Foods rich in GABA include bananas, citrus fruit, eggs, lentils, spinach, tomatoes, molasses, nuts, whole grains, seafood (halibut and shrimp), kefir, yogurt, and oolong and valerian root teas.

Practicing yoga increased GABA levels by about 27 percent compared to controls in a study at the Boston University of Medicine.[5] At the end of a long day, sitting on the couch and mindlessly watching hours of television may seem like the easy fix, but it doesn't bring peace and happiness. Instead, ditch the television and buy a yoga DVD, appropriate for your level of expertise, and accessories (mat, belt, and blocks). Start by performing some simple yoga poses for 10 minutes before bed. Slowly increase the time if you prefer.

GABA also comes in supplement form along with magnesium and vitamin B6, both essential for its utilization. GABA is frequently combined with other calming supplements. There are several good brands, including GABA Calm from Source Naturals and True Calm from Now Foods. See Appendix E for more details. Because these supplements have ingredients to relax and aid sleep, it is best to take them within an hour of bedtime.

NR20

Herbs That Calm

*Living a healthy lifestyle will only deprive you of poor
health, lethargy, and fat.*

~Jill Johnson

MANY HERBS ARE helpful for calming tremors. They are packaged as teas, liquid extracts, capsules, and tablets. Teas have weaker effects than the other forms. Below is a list of herbs recommended for treating Tremor. They are frequently combined with each other and with other supplements, such as GABA, for optimal effect. These herbs cause drowsiness, so it is best to take them before going to bed. In addition, taking them with alcohol or the drugs alprazolam, benzodiazepines, and other CNS sedatives may cause extreme drowsiness.

Chamomile

Because of its strong sedative and relaxing effect, herbalists recommend chamomile for inducing sleep and for calming hyperactive children. In one study, chamomile tea given to a group of twelve patients in a hospital put ten of them to sleep within 10 minutes.[1] Chamomile herbs are also effective for relief of diarrhea, flatulence, heartburn, and other digestive upsets.

Hops

Hops can treat anxiety, ADHD, insomnia, nervous tension, stress, low appetite, and menopausal hot flashes. Hops can prevent the formation of new blood vessels, so they may assist as an anticancer remedy. In one study, xanthohumol, a natural compound in hops, aided in preventing prostate cancer in men by blocking the effects of testosterone.[2] An animal study has shown that hops have a more positive effect on menopausal hot flashes than soy phytoestrogens.[3]

Passionflower

According to Medline, passionflower is a common treatment for insomnia, gastrointestinal upset related to anxiety or nervousness, generalized anxiety disorder, and relieving symptoms related to narcotic drug withdrawal. Passionflower also treats asthma, ADHD, seizures, hysteria, symptoms of menopause, nervousness and excitability, palpitations, irregular heartbeat, high blood pressure, fibromyalgia, and pain relief.[4]

Scientists are unsure why this herb is beneficial for anxiety, but they believe that passionflower increases GABA levels within the brain. In a study of 91 people with anxiety symptoms, researchers found that an herbal European product containing passionflower and other herbal sedatives significantly reduced symptoms of generalized anxiety compared to a placebo.[5]

Passionflower has performed as well as Oxazepam (a benzodiazepine) in reducing tremors influenced by anxiety in clinical studies. Generalized anxiety disorder impacts a considerable portion of people suffering from tremors that frequently goes unreported.

Skullcap

Skullcap is a nerve tonic effective for conditions of anxiety, excitability, insomnia, restlessness, and other nervous complaints. Skullcap has been used to heal physical irregularities like convulsions, epilepsy, heart trembles, and jerking muscles. Many holistic health experts have advocated the use of skullcap instead of antidepressants or tranquillizers to alleviate depression. The American Botanical Council reports that *King's American Dispensatory* recommends this herb to help treat tremors.[6]

Valerian

Valerian has an effect similar to benzodiazepine drugs but is weaker and without any of the potential side effects. It most commonly treats anxiety and insomnia but has also been used to calm nerves, treat depression, promote relaxation, and alleviate pain and headaches. Scientists are unsure why exactly this herb works, but suggest that, like passionflower, it enhances the relay of the GABA neurotransmitters in the body. Valerian is one of the most popular herbs used to treat tremors. It is frequently combined with hops, lemon balm, and/or skullcap. According to studies, skullcap improves the effectiveness of valerian root when they are taken together.

Alternative Therapies

NR21

Acupuncture

*So many people spend their health gaining wealth, and
then have to spend their wealth to regain their health.*

~A.J. Reb Materi

Acupuncture is one of the main forms of treatment in Traditional Chinese
Medicine (TCM). In TCM, disease is perceived as an imbalance of yin
and yang, or "qi." Yin and yang are opposing forces that must stay in balance. When they are out of balance, so is the health of the body. Qi, or
"chi," is the flow of energy in the body. When the body is in good health,
qi flows generously and smoothly. If qi is congested or blocked, disease
may result.

The goal of acupuncture is to restore the natural flow of energy along
the body's meridians, or energy pathways. To accomplish this, the practitioner inserts sharp, thin needles into the body at very specific points
called acupoints. The needles stimulate the central nervous system to
release the body's chemical messengers, hormones, and neurotransmitters. These chemicals boost the immune system, dull pain, and regulate

body functions. Advocates believe that the process adjusts and alters the body's energy flow into healthier patterns.

Acupuncture has been used in the treatment of allergies, arthritis, alcoholism and substance abuse, chronic pain, headaches, respiratory conditions, gastrointestinal disorders, gynecological problems, neurological disorders (including ET), and nervous conditions, plus childhood illnesses and disorders of the eyes, nose, and throat. In one study, acupuncture improved symptoms of ET by 59 percent. Of 60 people with ET, all were given medication, but half were also given acupuncture. Of those given the combination, 90 percent (27/30) improved compared to 56 percent (17/30) of the patients given the medication only.[1]

Acupressure is a technique similar to acupuncture. It uses the principles of acupuncture but stimulates acupoints with finger pressure instead of needles. Acupressure massage performed by a therapist, family member, or friend can be very effective to prevent and treat all of the health conditions that people use acupuncture to resolve. Acupuncture requires a visit to a professional, but anyone can perform acupressure. Its techniques are fairly easy to learn. All you need is a good instructional book or website on the topic.

NR22

Chiropractic

The brain forgets much, but the lower back remembers everything.

~Robert Brault

CHIROPRACTIC IS A form of alternative medicine that emphasizes diagnosis, treatment, and prevention of mechanical disorders of the musculoskeletal system with the belief that these disorders affect the general health of the nervous system. Daniel David Palmer, who founded chiropractic practices in 1895, believed that disease was the result of spinal bones that had become misaligned, especially those related to the central nervous system.

These misalignments (subluxations) of the spinal cord cause disease by interrupting the energy flow of specific nerves that send messages to related organs of the body. When energy flow is impaired to a particular body organ or part, dysfunction can result.

Chiropractors believe that there's a pattern to how ailments occur. First, the person has a misalignment of the spinal cord. Second, the person experiences pain in muscles or body structure. Third, the person has symptoms of nerve dysfunction that causes tingling, numbness, and/or pain. Lastly, the person's energy and health begin to fail. Some health conditions related to the misalignment of the spinal cord include breathing disorders such as asthma, cramps, headaches, and stomach ailments.

The basic chiropractic therapy is manual adjustment of what is distorted or misaligned with the body (spine or other skeletal bones). This realignment restores the normal positioning of the spine and structure of the body, which in turn relieves stress on the nervous system. When the nervous system is restored, energy can again flow correctly throughout the body, restoring and healing damaged or unhealthy body parts. Tense muscles can contribute to misalignment, so many chiropractors also utilize ultrasound and massage to help relax muscles.

Only one known study, using one person, has attempted to determine the effect of chiropractic treatments on ET. A 39-year-old woman was diagnosed with ET in 2000 and had had frequent migraine headaches with aura since the age of 10. She was given spinal manipulations in 2012. After just one manipulation, she showed improvement with both tremors and migraine headaches. The improvement remained after four months of treatment. Prior to treatment, she had tried several prescription and over-the-counter pain relievers for the migraines, with no relief.[1]

One person in one study certainly does not make for a definitive outcome. However, there is no need to wait for a double-blind study to try chiropractic. The price for chiropractic treatments is reasonable. The key is to find someone with good credentials and a good reputation. Ask family and friends for a referral or search the web for reviews, and make sure to check the chiropractor's credentials.

Those with a bone disease that causes weak or brittle bones and joints, such as osteoporosis, Paget's disease, or rheumatoid arthritis, should be extra cautious. Certain spinal manipulations could aggravate these conditions. Have your chiropractor consult with your primary care physician prior to treatment.

NR23

Homeopathy

It is easy to get a thousand prescriptions but hard to get one single remedy.

~CHINESE PROVERB

HOMEOPATHY IS A system of medicine that involves treatment with highly diluted substances, given mainly in tablet form, with the aim of triggering the body's natural system of healing. Samuel Hahnemann, who founded homeopathy in 1796, believed that a particular diluted substance that was in harmony with the "vital force" (also called chi or energy) would restore balance. Homeopathy remedies are created from animal, mineral, and plant substances diluted many times so that the original substance is virtually undetectable. Ironically, the more diluted a homeopathic remedy, the more potent it is, and the stronger its effect on symptoms.

The purpose of homeopathic remedies is to stimulate the mind and body to heal itself on all levels rather than to suppress symptoms the way conventional medicine can. Homeopathy is based on the principle of treating "like with like"—that is, a substance that in large doses causes symptoms can treat those symptoms with small doses. For example, drinking too much coffee can cause sleeplessness and agitation, so, according to this principle, a homeopathic coffee remedy (coffea cruda) can treat those symptoms. Conventional medicine sometimes uses this concept. For example, small doses of allergens such as pollen can desensitize people who are allergic to pollen. However, the major difference with homeopathic medicine is that its substances are in ultrahigh dilutions, which makes them nontoxic and completely safe.

Unlike traditional medicine, which provides a single medication for a condition, a single homeopathic remedy does not treat every person who has the same disease or medical condition. There are many possible remedies for any one condition, which behooves the practitioner to find the one that most accurately fits the client's symptoms, both physically and mentally. For instance, for a heartburn complaint, the practitioner needs to know about other symptoms. A wet cough accompanied by headaches, moodiness, and fatigue requires a different remedy than a dry cough accompanied by nausea and anxiety.

Unfortunately, there have been no studies on how homeopathic remedies affect ET, though a few studies have shown positive results for inflammatory-related conditions. In one, homeopathic and conventional treatments were combined to target periodontal disease. The result was more favorable than using conventional treatments alone.[1, 2] In another, homeopathy had positive effects on fibromyalgia.[3] In addition, a French study compared patients who went to general practitioners (GPs), who were certified in homeopathy, for URTI (upper respiratory tract infections) and those whose GPs were not. The patients of GPs certified in homeopathy used fewer antibiotics and antipyretic/anti-inflammatory drugs for URTI than patients of the completely conventional GPs.[4]

The main reason that few studies target holistic remedies is the lack of profit incentive for large pharmaceutical companies. Homeopathic remedies cost less than $10, on average, at nutritional-supplement stores. There is no need to pay for a trip to the doctor or expensive prescription drugs. In addition, classical homeopathy is based on individualized treatment, whereas most clinical research focuses on a single homeopathic remedy for all participants. As previously noted, the right remedy depends on the specific physical and emotional symptoms of an individual; otherwise, results are inaccurate.

Many scientists believe that homeopathic remedies work via the placebo effect. For some people, this may be true; however, holistic veterinarians have used homeopathic remedies to treat many animal ailments successfully, and animals are not subject to the placebo effect. In one pilot study, veterinarians submitted data regularly for 767 patients (547 dogs, 155 cats, 50 horses, 5 rabbits, 4 guinea pigs, 2 birds, 2 goats, 1 cow, and 1 tortoise). In 539 cases, the study obtained outcomes from two or more homeopathic appointments per patient condition. Out of those cases, 79.8 percent showed improvement, 11.7 percent had no change, and 6.1 percent showed deterioration. Follow-ups for 2.4 percent were not recorded. The strongest positive outcomes occurred in arthritis and epilepsy in dogs. Additional positive outcomes were in dermatitis, gingivitis, and hyperthyroidism in cats.[5]

Homeopathic remedies can work well with some modern medications. For example, homeopathic treatments have helped lessen the side effects of chemotherapy. However, modern medications can sometimes interfere with homeopathic remedies, rendering them inactive. The less medication taken alongside a homeopathic remedy, the higher the chance that the remedy will work as expected.

Homeopathic remedies come in many potencies and scales. The most common potencies available for sale are based on the C, or centesimal scale. A standard interval range of potencies for the C scale is 6C, 9C, 12C, 15C, 18C, 21C, 24C, 30C, 100C, 200C, and 500C. The higher the number on the scale, the more diluted the remedy and the higher the potency. Typical potencies sold at nutritional supplement stores are 6C, 12C, and 30C, but almost any of the above mentioned range of potencies can be found at online stores, such as Hahnemann Laboratories, Inc.

To make a remedy of 6C dilution, the homeopathic pharmacist takes one drop of the herbal tincture (called a mother tincture) and mixes it with 100 drops of water (with 20 percent solution of ethyl alcohol to act as a preservative). The solution is put in a vial and shook vigorously to obtain

1C of potency. Then the cycle is repeated by mixing one drop of the 1C with 100 drops of the solution to yield a potency of 2C. After 6 cycles of dilution and shaking vigorously, a dilution of 6C is produced.

Homeopaths believe Constantine Hering's "Law of Cure" is the basis of all healing. This theory is based on Hering's own observations of the order in which symptoms surface as part of the body's healing process. Symptoms improve from the top to bottom (relief is felt from upper to lower body parts) and from the deepest part (mental and emotional and vital organs such as the heart and lungs) to external parts (skin and extremities). They also appear and disappear in the reverse order of their original onset of appearance (from the most recent to the first symptoms).

Below is a list of commonly prescribed homeopathic remedies for tremors.[6, 7] Choose the best-matched remedy for your symptoms. Having all the symptoms for a particular remedy is not a requirement to have a match. It is best to start with one of the lower potencies, such as 3C or 6C. Signs of improvement may take a few days. Even if a remedy doesn't help your symptoms, it will not harm you either. If your symptoms improve, keep taking the remedy until you reach a plateau, then increase the dose. For example, if you start with a potency of 6C, increase to a potency of 9C or 12C. Keep doing this until symptoms are gone or the remedy stops working. Stop taking the remedy if symptoms disappear. If symptoms get worse or change, or the remedy stops working, you need a different remedy. Review symptoms again, and change to another remedy according to the new symptoms. A trained or certified homeopathic practitioner can save you time. Fees range from $30 to $80 per visit, depending on location, and usually require repeat visits to monitor progress.

1. **Agaricus Muscarius (fly agaric mushroom)**
    A remedy for twitching, jerking, trembling, and involuntary movements. Good for excessive tremors of hands, tongue, and head. May be chilly, even during warm weather. Symptoms are worse in cold weather and better in warm weather and evenings. Symptoms are worse when exhausted from mental activity, sex, or alcohol. Feels fearless but may have worries about cancer and

be preoccupied with death. Spasmodic sneezing and coughing (especially at night) may occur.

2. **Agentium Nitricum (silver nitrate)**
   Excellent remedy for those that have anxiety and nervous tension, along with tremors or trembling of the hands, tongue, or head. Might fear narrow places and crowds. Can be close to a nervous breakdown. Symptoms are worse when anticipating events or speaking engagements. Hoarse voice, especially after talking or singing. Symptoms are better in fresh, cool air and worse in warm weather.

3. **Cocculus Indicus (Indian cockle tree)**
   For tremors that affect one side of the body. Trembling from the slightest emotions or from noise, pains, or being touched. Very sensitive. Dislikes being disturbed and becomes angry when interrupted. Tends to feel faint and gets car- or seasickness easily. Symptoms worse after eating or loss of sleep and in the afternoon.

4. **Conium Maculatum (poison hemlock)**
   Good for trembling when accompanied by difficulty in walking and loss of strength. May have cysts or tumors, especially on breasts, ovaries, uterus, prostate, or testicles. Person becomes introverted. May withdraw emotionally and physically from others and become isolated. Often feels weak throughout entire body. Symptoms are worse when lying down, during menses, and with bodily or mental exertion.

5. **Gelsemium (yellow jasmine)**
   Recommended for those with shaking of hands worsened by anticipation and strong emotion. Dreads exams and suffers from stage fright. Fear of losing control. Onset of symptoms is slow and may be triggered by an emotional upset or shock. Accompanied by weakness and drowsiness. Knees tremble when walking downhill or downstairs. Symptoms are worse in hot, summer heat and before thunderstorms. Has lack of thirst during the heat.

6. **Lachesis (bushmaster snake)**
   For excessive shaking that is generally on the left side of the body. Also, for shaking that accompanies menopause. Has an

overactive mind. Talkative and tends to jump from one subject to the next. Passionate about life. May experience a sensation of suffocation when lying down or a dry fitful cough. Heart palpitations at menopause (male and female). Poor circulation and varicose veins. Symptoms are worse on waking.

7. **Mercurius Vivus (mercury)**

   For tremors that seem to be everywhere (inside and out) and occur with the least exertion. May have swollen glands and suffer from ulcerative colitis. Has intense thirst for cold drinks and continuous hunger. Conservative in nature and abides by a strict moral code. Has poor memory and willpower, lacks confidence, and is indecisive. Symptoms are worse at night and when lying on the right side.

8. **Plumbum Metallicum (lead)**

   For treating tremors of the hands that are accompanied by muscular weakness in arms and legs. This is a good remedy for also treating tremors in MS. May have pains in muscles of thighs and cramps in calves. Paralysis of the muscles or progressive muscle atrophy is common. May have partial or total loss of memory, depression, or fear of being killed. Symptoms are worse at night and better from rubbing with hard pressure and from physical exertion.

9. **Zincum Metallicum (zinc)**

   For trembling of the hands and head accompanied by weakness, trembling, and twitching of various muscles. Varicose veins, especially of lower limbs. May have restless feet. Ravenous hunger with poor digestion and constipation. Very sensitive to noise. Exhausted emotionally and physically. Complains constantly and can't let go of things that bother them. Symptoms worse with alcohol and cannot tolerate wine.

—ᚚ—

Below are guidelines for taking homeopathic remedies. They are vibrational medicine, which can be easily overwhelmed by other strong material vibrations. Be sure to follow these guidelines; they are essential for success.

- Remedies usually come in small vials. If a homeopathic practitioner prescribed them, follow his or her instructions. *It is important NOT to touch the pellets with your hand or fingers or place them on a counter or in another container first.* Place one to two pellets in the vial lid either by turning the lid upside down and pressing or by carefully dropping one or two pellets into it. Some containers allow direct placement into the mouth by pressing on the lid over the mouth. Place the pellets directly under your tongue and let them dissolve there for best absorption.
- Sunlight, moisture, heat, and strong odors can inactivate homeopathic remedies. Store them in a cool, dry, dark place. Avoid exposing them to moisture, temperatures above 120° F, and all strong odors.
- Do not take the remedy while outside or near a window in direct sunlight.
- Do not eat, drink, or use toothpaste for 30 minutes before or after taking the remedy. A good time to take it would be right before bed, as long as it is at least 30 minutes after you've had your evening meal and brushed your teeth.
- Do not drink any type of coffee while taking homeopathic remedies at any time of the day. The acid in the coffee is an antidote that may prevent the remedy from working.
- Do not use products containing camphor, such as Bengay, Blistex, Campho-Phenique, Noxzema, Tiger Balm, Carmex, Vicks, or anything that smells like them. These products deactivate the remedy.
- Do not use mint-flavored (spearmint, peppermint, wintermint, etc.) products such as toothpaste, gum, or candy. The mint deactivates the remedy.
- Do not get any dental work that involves drilling, grinding, or ultrasonic cleaning while taking homeopathic remedies. The products used in these procedures deactivate the remedy.
- Do not place homeopathic remedies in close contact with magnets.

NR24

Meditation

Meditation is a way for nourishing and blossoming the divinity within you.

~AMIT RAY

MEDITATION IS A practice in which an individual trains the mind to realize some benefit. It comprises a broad variety of practices that include techniques designed to promote relaxation, build internal energy, or life force, and develop compassion, love, patience, generosity, and forgiveness. Most meditative techniques began as part of Eastern religious traditions for attaining higher spiritual goals. Many different cultures throughout the world have used them for thousands of years. Today, many people use meditation outside of its traditional religious or cultural settings. Millions of Americans currently practice some form of meditation, including NFL football players, US Marines, and many famous people—Jennifer Aniston, Halle Berry, Kobe Bryant, Sheryl Crowe, Richard Gere, Paul McCartney, Rupert Murdoch, Katy Perry, Sting, and Oprah Winfrey.

Research findings on the positive effects of meditation show that it can offer all of the following benefits:

- Improved mental activity related to attention, learning, and conscious perception
- Boosted immunity with increased antibodies
- Reduced inflammation and pain
- Increased ability to focus
- Feelings of emotional well-being and life satisfaction
- Improved memory with increased gray matter in the brain
- Reduced depression, anxiety, and stress

Anxiety and stress present challenges for most people, but they are particularly troublesome for people with Tremor. During stress, the body releases the neurochemical adrenaline that aggravates tremors. Any method of reducing the effect of stress on the body and limiting the effects of adrenaline is beneficial. Neuroscientists have found that when people meditate, they shift their brain activity to different areas of the cortex. Brain waves in the stress-prone right frontal cortex move to the calmer left frontal cortex. This mental shift decreases the negative effects of mild depression, anxiety, and stress.[1]

Although no clinical research has investigated the effects of meditation on the shaking of ET, Dr. Elan D. Louis, professor of neurology and epidemiology at Columbia University, says that meditation may help: "Stress and anxiety can certainly temporarily exacerbate an underlying tremor disorder. To my knowledge, it has not been rigorously tested whether stress reduction through meditation temporarily lessens Tremor. That is, I know of no clinical trials. However, meditation could, at least in theory, provide some mild temporary reduction in Tremor."[2]

Techniques for meditating include mantra, relaxation-response, mindfulness, and Zen Buddhist meditation. Meditation practices focus one's awareness or attention, often through the repetition of a word, sound, or phrase, or just through breathing.

Meditation does not have to take a significant amount of time or space. A comfortable and quiet place to sit and a timer is all you need. Start with 10 minutes. Set the timer and either chant a mantra or pay attention to your breathing. It's difficult to stop the mind from drifting initially. Don't worry. With practice, it becomes easier to stay focused.

Part IV

Putting It All Together

A Personalized Step-by-Step Guide

It is better to make many small steps in the right direction than to make a great leap forward only to stumble.

~PROVERB

CONGRATULATIONS! YOU JUST finished reading just about anything you can find in medical journals, books, or on the Internet about ET and tremors in general. Now that I've saved you months of time, what do you do with all this information? Below is a step-by-step guide to help you put together a personalized plan. Step 1 starts with a set of questions to help narrow down the cause or trigger of your tremors. Step 2 lists medical tests to take based on your answers in Step 1. Steps 3 through 7 cover the natural remedies discussed in Part III in a concise format, with references to the appropriate chapters so that you can easily go back and review the material.

Step 1: Determining the cause(s) of your tremors

Answer whether the following statements are true or false:

1. You eat wheat products (except ancient grains like spelt or einkorn) every day and feel you can't live without them. NR1
2. You eat genetically engineered food (nonorganic soy, corn, cottonseed oil, and beet sugar) daily. NR1
3. You drink diet soft drinks several times per week. NR2
4. You eat Chinese takeout and packaged soups several times per week. NR2
5. You use primarily canola and vegetable oils for cooking or frying. NR3
6. You eat a low-fat diet. NR3
7. You eat lots of processed and nonorganic meats. NR4
8. Your favorite way to cook meat is grilling. NR4
9. You have a sweet tooth and must consume something sweet at almost every meal. NR5
10. You eat, on average, two or fewer servings of fruits and vegetables a day, excluding ketchup and French fries. NR5
11. You frequently feel stressed or depressed. NR6
12. You are not very happy with your job, partner or spouse, parents, children, or friendships. NR6
13. You have irregular sleep patterns, trouble falling asleep, or trouble sleeping through the night. NR7
14. You are a woman over 40 and have hot flashes, night sweats, fatigue, trouble sleeping, moodiness, or dry skin and hair. NR8
15. You are frequently hyperactive and unable to gain weight, or you have problems losing weight with diet and exercise. NR8
16. You have a low libido, brain fog, forgetfulness, or memory problems. NR8, NR9
17. You regularly take drugs to treat anxiety, congestion, depression, high blood pressure, hyperactivity, low thyroid, mood disorders, or seizures. NR9

18. You drink coffee, liquor, beer, or wine in excess, and/or smoke cigarettes or marijuana. NR9
19. You get little sun exposure and do not take a vitamin D supplement. NR10
20. You have a chronic health problem that you are aware of, such as arthritis, diabetes, gum disease, heart disease, Crohn's disease, IBD, or osteoporosis. Appendixes A, B, and D
21. You use wireless technology, including a smart phone, wireless computer or tablet, or video-game consoles for several hours each day. NR11
22. You have a smart meter within 30 feet of your bedroom. NR11
23. You live within approximately 1,200 feet, or about a quarter mile, from a cell tower or power plant. NR11
24. You love to garden and use chemical herbicides or pesticides to keep weeds or bugs away. NR12
25. You mainly use household cleaners with chemical additives instead of natural products. NR12
26. You recently moved into a newly-built house or work in a newly-remodeled office with synthetic carpet, particleboard flooring, particleboard cabinets, or new pressed-wood furniture. NR12
27. Your house was built prior to 1977 and you removed the paint from the walls yourself without protective gear. NR13
28. You have many dental fillings made from amalgam. NR13, Appendix B
29. You work closely with toxic metals in the mining, welding, painting, plastics, or chemical industry. NR13
30. You get the flu vaccine every year without fail. NR14

Step 2: Diagnostic tests to rule out medical reasons for your tremors
Basic tests are important to rule out any medical reasons for your tremors regardless of your answers in Step 1. These should include blood tests, urine tests, and an EMG. Blood tests should consist of a CMP, CBC, CRP, and thyroid panel. Urine tests should consist of a urinalysis and heavy

metal screening. An EMG helps differentiate between PD and ET tremors by measuring electrical activity in the muscles.

Then, based on your answers in Step 1, add the following tests:

- Hemoglobin A1c: Averages your blood sugar over the past two to three months. If you answered True for 1, 3, 6, 9, 16, or 20 or are prediabetic or diabetic.
- Vitamin B12: If you are a vegan or answered True for 16.
- Magnesium: If you answered True for 3, 9, 10, 13, 18, 19, or 20.
- Vitamin D: If you answered True for 18, 19, or 20.
- LDL particle test (NMR Lipid Profile, or NMR lipoprofile): If you answered True for 1, 2, 5, 6, 9, or 10 or have heart disease. This test measures the size of LDL particle number. According to LabCorp, the goal for someone with heart disease, diabetes or other high risk condition is an optimum LDL particle number under 1,000. The goal for everyone else is 1,000-1,299 and is considered near or above optimum, 1,300-1,599 is borderline high, 1,600-2,000 is high and over 2,000 is very high.
- Toxic metals: Test for lead if you answered True for 27, drank water from lead pipes, or used garden hoses that were not lead-free to grow food. Test for mercury if you answered True for 28 and 30. Test for aluminum if you answered True for 30, used aluminum cookware, or drank from aluminum cans regularly. Test for manganese if you worked as a welder or miner. Test for copper if you drank from copper pipes or suspect Wilson's disease.
- Progesterone, estrogen, and testosterone levels: If you answered True for 14 and 16 and you are a woman.
- Testosterone and estrogen levels: If you are a man over the age of 40, check your testosterone levels. If you are overweight (especially if you have man boobs) or answered True for 24, 25, or 29, get your estrogen levels checked, too. Men have estrogen that can become elevated from xenoestrogens (artificial estrogens) in the environment.

- Imaging tests: MRI, CT scan, and/or X-rays if you have unresolved headaches, sleep problems, memory loss, or another medical condition for which your doctor recommends imaging tests.

Step 3: Clean up your diet

Get rid of all frankenfoods and junk food. This includes processed foods with lists of chemical ingredients and anything that contains aspartame, MSG, HFCS, nonorganic soy and corn, canola, and hydrogenated fats. Look at the ingredients in frozen meals, boxed cereals, canned foods, and sauces or salad dressings. Most salad dressings are made with hydrogenated fats and lots of HFCS or sugar. Also, throw out anything that has sugar as one of the first three ingredients. Buy raw honey, pure maple syrup, and stevia for sweeteners and organic butter, coconut oil, and olive oil to replace the unhealthy oils. Buy sea salt, ground pepper, mustard, turmeric, garlic powder, curry powder, chili powder, basil, and other herbs and spices to make food taste great so you won't be tempted to run out for fast food.

Make your own soups, salads, and salad dressings. Stock up on plenty of fresh and frozen fruits and vegetables, nuts (almonds, walnuts, Brazil nuts, cashews, and pine nuts), seeds (sunflower, pumpkin, and sesame), legumes (beans, lentils, and peas), nut butters (almond, cashew, and peanut), and whole grains (brown rice, buckwheat, millet, oats, and quinoa). Unless you are going gluten free, you can pick up some whole grain, low-gluten flours (spelt, barley, and oat). For baking, use aluminum-free baking powder, like Rumford.

For protein, eat organic tofu, organic eggs, hormone-free yogurt, and free-range organic chicken. Eat grass-fed beef and wild-caught fish in moderation. Check back to the *Food Choices* section for more details on diet.

For those who want to try going gluten free, get rid of everything in your house with gluten in it. Purchase some gluten-free flour mixes or mix your own from any combination of almond, buckwheat, oat (must state gluten free on the package), potato, sorghum, tapioca, teff, or quinoa flours. Bob's Red Mill sells a great-tasting, gluten-free, all-purpose flour mix. For baking, you also need xanthan gum (substitute for gluten), aluminum-free baking powder, and baking soda. Many great gluten-free recipes can be found on the Internet and in books from your local library.

Step 4: Clean up your life

The following are necessary steps for eliminating lifestyle triggers of your tremors.

A. Work to resolve chronic stress or depression. Figure out what you don't like about your life. Making one small change toward your goals frequently lifts depression. Make a commitment to yourself to make one change at a time. If you don't like your job or career, investigate a new one. Work with a life or career coach if you can afford it. Life is too short to be unhappy. If you are not exercising, start a program that you enjoy. There is no better way to reduce stress and depression.

B. Resolve any sleep issues. Review NR7.

C. Take hormone replacement based on laboratory test results, if needed. In the meantime, women can try an over-the-counter natural progesterone cream or maca root. Low testosterone does not typically cause tremors, but it does cause other health issues. Sex hormone levels can also be boosted naturally by exercising, taking zinc and vitamin D (or getting sun exposure), and avoiding endocrine disruptors, which lower hormone levels and increase cancer risk. Review NR8 and NR12.

D. Research any drugs you are taking for side effects of shaking or tremors. If any of them could cause or trigger tremors, see your doctor immediately for a replacement. Review NR9.

E. If you are taking cholesterol-lowering drugs, cleaning up your diet can reduce inflammation and cholesterol levels. Make sure you are taking CoQ10 if you are taking statins. Then work with your doctor to decrease your dependence on them. Follow the recommendations for heart health in Appendix D.

Step 5: Clean up your environment

The following are necessary steps for reducing environmental triggers of your tremors.

   A. Reduce the number of wireless devices in your house by getting rid of what is not essential and wiring everything else that can be wired. Make sure there is no turned-on wireless device or electrical device within five feet of your bed while sleeping. Review NR11.

   B. Replace all chemical household cleaning products with natural alternatives. Review NR12.

   C. Determine if you are exposed to any toxic metals in your home or work life. If so, block the exposure or remove it. If you are exposed at work, then staying there is risking your health. Decide what is more important. Review NR13.

   D. Decide whether vaccinations are worth the risks. Work on building natural immunity. Review NR14.

Step 6: Add nutritional supplements

The following supplements are important for controlling symptoms of ET. Start with the supplements in A and work through to E as funds permit. See Appendix E for more details and dosage recommendations.

   A. Take a quality MVM, B-complex, and magnesium supplement. Add extra B12 if you are a vegan or have mood or memory problems. Add extra vitamin D if you tested low or deficient. Review NR10, NR16, and NR18.

   B. If you are not eating fermented foods, add probiotics. If you are not eating raw foods, add digestive enzymes. Review Appendix A.

   C. Add a calming supplement that contains GABA and calming herbs. Review NR19 and NR20.

   D. Add a choline supplement, especially if you have brain fog or forgetfulness. Review NR17.

E. Add as many antioxidants as your budget permits. Choose those that are appropriate for your symptoms and budget except for one exception—CoQ10. It is a must for anyone on cholesterol-lowering drugs or over the age of 40. Review NR15.

Step 7: Add an alternative therapy

About three months after completing Step 6, add an alternative therapy (acupuncture, acupressure, chiropractic, homeopathy, or meditation) that fits your budget and lifestyle. Give each therapy at least two months before switching to or adding a different one. Don't try more than one at a time, because if your symptoms improve, you won't know which therapy worked. Review the *Alternative Therapies* section.

APPENDIX A

Importance of Digestive Aids

The road to health is paved with good intestines!

~Sherry A. Rogers

Digestive aids are substances that help break down food and support the health of the digestive tract. They enable the body to absorb and use nutrients properly. Digestive enzymes and probiotics are the two main types of digestive aids. Without sufficient amounts of these substances, the body does not obtain all the potential nutrients in food.

Americans take large amounts of prescription and over-the-counter drugs to try to solve digestive problems, like laxatives for constipation. Medications not only mask the problems, but they frequently make matters worse. Having less than one bowel movement a day is a sign of chronic constipation. Over time, chronic constipation results in the compromised integrity of the bowel. Antigens, substances that create an immune response, form and permeate the gut wall to leak into the lymphatic and circulatory systems, producing an inflammatory immune response that can lead to increased infections and many chronic conditions including arthritis, asthma, depression, eczema, fibromyalgia, food allergies, IBD, irritability, loss of concentration and memory, and psoriasis.

Abdominal gas, bloating, heartburn, diarrhea, and frequent infections are more signs of inadequate digestion. Digestive aids can help solve these problems and constipation without drugs.

Digestive enzymes
Digestive enzymes are complex protein molecules that aid in the digestive process by breaking down food into particles small enough to pass through the walls of the small intestine to the blood. Some digestive

enzymes are produced in our bodies, and some come from food. The different types of digestive enzymes are called amylase, protease, and lipase. Amylase helps in digesting carbohydrates. It helps reduce bloating and gas by helping digest sugars found in legumes and vegetables. Amylase reduces carbohydrates to disaccharides called lactose, maltose, and sucrose. These molecules are further broken down by specific enzymes that the small intestine makes. Lactase helps in the digestion of dairy products and lactose. Maltase and sucrase help in the digestion of starches and sugars. Protease and lipase help in digesting proteins and fats, respectively.

Digestion occurs in stages. It begins in the mouth with chewing. When food is chewed thoroughly, the salivary glands secrete the enzyme amylase, which begins the breakdown of carbohydrates. Swallowed food enters the upper part of the stomach and waits for 30 to 60 minutes for the body to produce pepsin and hydrochloric acid (HCl) to activate enzymes for protein digestion. Food then moves down the stomach into the small intestine. This food, called chyme, sends a hormonal signal to the pancreas, informing it of how much protein, carbohydrate, and fat is left to be digested. The pancreas secretes enzymes to complete the job.

Raw foods, including raw fruits and vegetables, are loaded with enzymes. Cooking food at temperatures over 118 degrees destroys them. The average American consumes significantly less raw food than our ancestors did 60 to 70 years ago before processed and fast foods became very popular. People who follow a raw food diet today know the importance of enzymes. Ideally, a diet of 50 percent raw food would supply all the enzymes most people need. Most of us have difficulty even doing that, especially in the winter months. That's why digestive enzyme supplements are important. But for those suffering from disorders that were a result of poor digestion or whose conditions contributed to poor digestion, enzyme supplementation is essential. Good candidates for supplementation are those suffering from allergies, celiac disease, constipation, GERD or heartburn, gallstones, IBS, low energy, pancreatitis, and any chronic condition, including Tremor. Lipase enzymes are especially important for those who've had a cholecystectomy, or their gallbladder removed. The gallbladder's main function is to store bile secreted by the liver and use it to emulsify fats. Without a gallbladder, a supplement with lipase is needed to aid fat digestion and should be taken with every meal that contains fat.

A typical enzyme supplement contains papain (papaya) or bromelain (pineapple) to digest protein, amylase to break down carbohydrates, and lipase to break down fats. It can also contain lactase for breaking down lactose found in dairy products. Enzyme supplements come from animal and plant sources. Animal sources of digestive enzymes come from the pancreas (pancreatin) of pigs and the gallbladder (ox-bile extract) of oxen. Animal-based enzymes are not as efficient for aiding digestion in the stomach as compared to plant-based digestive enzymes. However, pancreatin may be helpful for those with pancreatitis or pancreatic cancer and ox-bile extract may be helpful for those with liver or gallbladder problems. Plant-based enzymes come from fruit or aspergillus oryzae, a fungus grown in a lab on a plant medium. Aspergillus helps in the digestion of food starting in the stomach, thus making them more effective than other enzyme sources for reducing stress on the intestines. Aspergillus is the best overall for vegans and those with symptoms of heartburn, flatulence, and constipation.

Probiotics

Probiotics, also called gut flora, are microorganisms (intestinal bacteria) that help keep the intestines healthy by allowing nutrients to easily pass into the bloodstream. The beneficial bacteria keep the dangerous ones, like C. difficile, in check by competing with them for food and pushing them out of places to hang out and multiply. Probiotics also produce a mild acetic solution, which is toxic to harmful bacteria.

Probiotics not only improve digestion, they reduce constipation, boost immunity, regulate hormones, lower cholesterol, reduce risk of certain cancers, and relieve symptoms of IBS and yeast infections. Good candidates for probiotics are those who suffer from belly fat, constipation, flatulence, and frequent colds and infections.

Fermented foods or supplements can supply probiotics. A daily serving of any one of the following foods will help build gut flora. It's best to vary them each day to maximize benefits.

- **Sauerkraut and pickles.** These products should be refrigerated and not pasteurized. If they are not refrigerated, they do not contain live bacteria. The bacteria in pasteurized products are also dead.
- **Miso, tofu, natto, and tempeh.** These products should be refrigerated and organic. Most (90 percent or more) of nonorganic soy comes from plants that are genetically modified and heavily sprayed with herbicides. Use organic tamari or shoyu instead of soy sauce with these foods. Both contain live bacteria and no GMOs.
- **Fermented dairy products.** Yogurt, kefir, and cottage cheese are all fermented. Organic kefir, a fermented dairy drink, tastes like drinkable yogurt. Purchase those made without artificial hormones and check the label for active cultures.

The most effective probiotic supplement should include L. acidophilus and B. bifidum in addition to any combination of the following: L. salivarius, L. bulgaricus, L. casei, B. infantis, B. brevis, B. longum, Bacillus coagulans, and S. thermophilus. (L. refers to lactobacillus, B. refers to bifidobacteria, and S. refers to streptococcus). Look for products that contain at least one billion bacteria per serving.

If you must take antibiotics, adding probiotics during and after is important because antibiotics indiscriminately kill off *all* bacteria living in the intestines, good and bad. This is why many women commonly develop yeast infections after taking them. A little preventative planning can save another trip to the doctor or hospital. Hospitals can be high-risk zones for acquiring infections with the rise in superbugs. If you do visit the hospital for any reason, it's wise to take additional probiotics before you go.

APPENDIX B

Importance of Good Oral Hygiene

I've been to the dentist several times so I know the drill.

~Anonymous

Periodontal disease, the scientific name for all gum disease from gingivitis to periodontitis, has been linked to many chronic conditions, including heart disease, Alzheimer's, diabetes, and strokes. Gingivitis is inflammation and swelling of the gums. Periodontitis is the last stage of periodontal disease, when the ligaments that attach a tooth to bone are inflamed and infected, as well as the bone itself. Periodontitis results in tooth loss if not resolved.

According to the mainstream dental experts, periodontal disease is a result of poor dental hygiene. It starts with tartar formation on teeth from bacteria due to improper brushing and flossing. Failing to go to the dentist to get the tartar removed results in gum infection. As the infection spreads below the gum line, pockets form between the gums and the teeth, causing the gum line to recede. In time, the infection breaks down bone and connective tissues until the teeth become loose and fall out or need to be extracted.

Some people brush their teeth religiously yet still end up with gingivitis. There are other factors besides poor dental hygiene that can contribute to bacterial buildup in the mouth. Hormonal changes in the body, medications that cause dry mouth, bacteria spreading in the body, and diabetes can all play a part in developing gingivitis.

About 70 years ago, Weston Price studied isolated populations who did not practice oral hygiene but were free of tooth decay and gum disease. These indigenous people, however, ate only healthy, whole foods.[1] They had no access to highly-processed foods. But when they were introduced to the Western diet, dental disease followed. The diets of the people studied by Weston Price were alkaline. The Western diet is much more acidic. Acid helps accelerate tooth decay. Overall, Western diets do not support good health. In a healthy body, bad bacteria, infections, and disease are minimal.

If you have sore, sensitive teeth, sore gums, gingivitis, or periodontal disease, you need to make some changes. The following recommendations will help improve not only the health of your mouth, but your overall health as well.

1. **Avoid fast-food restaurants and processed foods.**
   This includes anything with artificial ingredients, colorings, flavorings, preservatives, GMOs, and chemicals with multisyllabic names. These foods are likely to have an acidic pH that promotes tartar.

2. **Limit dairy.**
   Your teeth are bones. Bone-fracture rates are highest in countries that consume the most dairy, calcium, and animal protein. As mentioned in NR9, there is little evidence that milk or other dairy products benefit bones. Consume no more than two servings (8 ounces of yogurt or 1 ounce of cheese equal one serving) of plain yogurt and aged or raw cheeses daily.

3. **Eat a salad every day.**
   Vegetables are alkaline. Eating a raw salad with a minimum of four vegetables every day provides you with lots of digestive enzymes, antioxidants, vitamins, and minerals. Good food choices for a salad include romaine lettuce, spinach, avocados, apples slices, pineapple, cabbage, cucumbers, carrots, peppers, tomatoes, radishes, and red onions. For protein, you can add cooked legumes such as chickpeas or kidney beans or a small amount of organic grilled chicken (Keep in mind that all meat is acidic). Try not to eat the same salad with the same ingredients everyday. Every fruit and vegetable has different nutrients so variety is important. Make your own salad dressing from olive oil, vinegar, garlic powder, basil, sea salt, and pepper. Distilled vinegar is

typically made from GM corn. Apple cider and balsamic vinegars are better choices. Lemon juice can be substituted for vinegar.

4. **Take digestive enzymes.**

Enzymes boost digestion of nutrients from food, which helps keep teeth and gums strong and healthy. We lose enzymes as we age. If you eat raw salads every day, you may not need a supplement. Keep a supply for days you don't eat raw produce. In the winter, my family eats more soups than salads so we take them every day.

5. **Eat plenty of healthy fats.**

Better, more alkaline fats come from coconut, olive, and avocado oils. Organic butter is good in moderation. Fats from red meats, vegetable oils, and trans-fatty acids are too acidic.

6. **Eliminate refined sugar, white flour, and white rice.**

White flour and white rice act like sugar in the body. Brown sugar is no better. It is just white, refined sugar with molasses added. Sugar feeds bacterial infections, so it must be eliminated or severely limited, or your gums will keep deteriorating. Sugar causes cavities due to its acidic nature in the body rather than because it is on the teeth. Brushing your teeth cannot remove the acidic effect of sugar, or an acidic diet, from your body. In general, most processed foods and animal products (dairy, fish, and meat) are acid-promoting, and most fruits and vegetables are alkaline-promoting. A diet that is 60 to 80 percent alkaline is ideal.

7. **Take supplements that support bone health.**

Magnesium and vitamins A, B, C, D, and E are essential to good dental health. The vitamins can be taken together in a quality MVM. A separate magnesium supplement is needed.

8. **Stop smoking.**

Smoking cigarettes or marijuana depresses the immune system and introduces free radicals and other toxins that damage the gums, thereby promoting the growth of harmful bacteria. They also stain your teeth. Chewing-tobacco products are even worse. It's like injecting the toxins directly into your gums.

9. **Gently brush your teeth and gums after eating.**

   Change your toothbrush every month if you have receding gums or gingivitis and at least every three months when the infection clears up. Use natural toothpaste made without chemicals and fluoride. Fluoride promotes dental fluorosis, which can weaken bones and teeth, allowing cavities and discoloration to form.

10. **Drink plenty of water.**

    Water is a natural detoxifier. Drink 8 to 12 cups of filtered, fluoride-free water daily, depending on your size and activity level.

11. **Take a garlic supplement.**

    Garlic inhibits microbial growth due to allicin, a sulfur-based compound. This compound can be used to inhibit the growth of bacteria as well as fungal growth in the mouth and body.[2] A good-quality and odorless garlic supplement is Kyolic.

12. **Add oil pulling with coconut oil to your daily routine.**

    Coconut oil kills bacteria. It gets between the teeth more thoroughly than brushing, flossing, and gargling with mouthwash. To oil pull, put a spoonful of coconut oil into your mouth and swish it around for 10 to 15 minutes. It will suck up bacteria, toxins, pus, and mucus. After you're done, spit it in the trash or a container. Spitting the oil into your sink may clog it up over time. Don't swallow the oil, or you'll deposit bacteria into your body.

13. **Chew gum or drink lemon juice with honey for dry mouth.**

    Certain medications can cause gum disease by decreasing the body's production of saliva. Saliva helps keep teeth clean and inhibit bacterial growth. Common drugs that suppress the salivary glands include anticholinergics, antidepressants, cold remedies, antihistamines, anticonvulsants, blood-pressure drugs, and immunosuppressants.[3] All of these drugs can also cause memory problems, so you get to lose your teeth and memory at the same time. Among the most potent salivary gland inhibitors are anticholinergics, which are used for muscle-control problems and to balance dopamine and acetylcholine levels. They are commonly used to treat depression, incontinence, and insomnia. Work with a holistic healthcare practitioner to reduce dependence on drugs. Until then, be extremely diligent with oral hygiene and try stimulating the salivary glands naturally by chewing gum and drinking lemon juice with a little raw honey.

14. **Go to the dentist for regular check ups.**

    Finally, go to the dentist for regular cleanings and take care of existing dental problems. During cleanings, dental hygienists frequently cause minor tears in gums, leading to bleeding. Even that can spread bacteria, so immediately following any dental procedure, take garlic supplements and oil pull to reduce the chance of bacteria spreading. If the dentist gives you antibiotics, make sure to take probiotics as well to replace the good bacteria that the antibiotics are destroying.

APPENDIX C

Importance of Exercise

*Those who think they have not time for bodily exercise
will sooner or later have to find time for illness.*

~Edward Stanley

Physical activity stimulates neuron growth, which is needed for learning, cognitive function, and movement. At some point, neurons become dysfunctional and die. When new neurons can't keep up with dying neurons, physical and mental functions decline, resulting in cognitive impairment and all neurodegenerative conditions.[1]

Scientists used to believe that we were born with a certain number of brain neurons and that the number could only decline. Recent studies have shown that neuron growth can be stimulated through exercise. In one study, researchers found that the creation of new neuron cells in the brain dropped off dramatically in middle-aged mice compared with younger ones, but that exercise significantly slowed the loss of nerve cells in the middle-aged mice. In addition, production of new brain cells in the mice that exercised increased by approximately 200 percent compared to the middle-aged mice that did not.[2] What this study means is that exercise is critical for proper brain function through all of life.

There is no proof that lack of exercise causes Tremor. However, since exercise slows the loss of brain neurons and stimulates the production of new ones, it may very well slow or prevent the progression of tremors in ET. Below is a list of the many benefits of exercise. *Everyone* should exercise, but for those with a neurological condition, it's imperative. Seek your doctor's approval before starting an exercise program, especially if you have been leading a sedentary lifestyle or have a serious, chronic condition.

1. **Stimulates brain-neuron growth and slows loss of existing neurons.**
   This is the number one reason for anyone with ET to put some movement into their life.
2. **Improves mood and lifts depression.**
   Dealing with a chronic condition can affect mood and lead to depression. Physical activity increases production of endorphins, the feel-good hormones. Exercising is the best antidepressant that exists, and you don't need a prescription from your doctor or time for psychological counseling.
3. **Boosts energy.**
   Exercise aids in the delivery of oxygen and nutrients to your tissues. Exercise helps you get the most from the money you spend on healthy food and nutritional supplements.
4. **Enhances quality of sleep.**
   Moving your body a few hours before bedtime helps you fall asleep faster and sleep deeper. People who don't sleep well have higher risk of tremors and dementia.
5. **Strengthens bones.**
   All exercise, but especially weight-bearing exercise, builds bone tissue. It can even reverse osteoporosis.
6. **Increases strength.**
   Exercise builds muscle mass. Frailty is associated with increased tremors, so stay strong.
7. **Improves circulation and reduces blood pressure.**
   High blood pressure and poor blood circulation increase risk of anxiety and symptoms of shaking.
8. **Reduces risk of chronic conditions.**
   Exercise reduces the risk of developing diabetes and death from cardiovascular disease in those with diabetes.[3, 4]
9. **Lowers risk of falling by increasing flexibility.**
   Flexibility increases through elongating muscles, such as in stretching or yoga.

10. Improves self-confidence.
Achieving improvement milestones and a more toned body are self-esteem builders.

11. Slows aging.
The cells of people who exercise look younger than those who are sedentary, according to one study.[5] In addition, it reduces overall stress levels. Stress has been linked to premature aging.[6]

12. Lowers risk of colon and breast cancers.[7, 8]
Exercise is a natural laxative. It keeps the digestive system moving along, getting toxins out of the body quicker.

13. Reduces inflammation.
Even relatively modest physical activity has proven to reduce inflammatory biomarkers (results of CRP tests). This may be due to exercise's positive effect on energy, mood, sleep, and stress levels.

An exercise program should consist of a combination of strength training, aerobics, and stretching. Strength training is any activity that builds muscles. Do it for 30 minutes, two to three times per week, alternating between upper and lower body. Start out slow, with the lightest weight that gives you some resistance. Injury is easy when you don't perform moves properly, so if you have never used free weights or resistance equipment, employ a personal trainer for your first 10 to 12 sessions; it is time and money well spent. Other strength-training options include cross-country skiing, stair climbing with dumbbells in hands, or performing yoga poses. Floor exercises such as sit-ups, push-ups, and lunges also build muscle.

Stretching is important for keeping joints flexible. Tai chi movements or yoga poses are a good way to combine stretching and strength training. Tai chi strengthens the abs, back, and upper and lower body, in addition to relieving pain. Yoga increases flexibility and strength, in addition to relieving stress and expanding mindfulness. Start with 10 minutes and work up to 30, three times per week.

Aerobics strengthen the cardiovascular system, which is important for keeping the heart healthy and the blood flowing. Blood carries nutrients and oxygen throughout the body, including to the brain to nourish neurons. Aerobic activities include jogging, swimming, cross-country skiing, biking, dancing, and power, or speed, walking. Do one for at least 30 minutes and at least three times per week. Aerobics for 10 minutes, three times per day, is even more effective. All you need is a good pair of athletic shoes and 10 minutes after each meal. You can walk (outside or on a treadmill), dance, jump on a mini trampoline, jump rope, or ride a bicycle (stationary or moving).

APPENDIX D

Inflammation and Chronic Disease

First the doctor told me the good news. I was going to have a disease named after me.

~STEVE MARTIN

Inflammation is associated with every chronic condition including heart disease, diabetes, depression, neurodegeneration, rheumatoid arthritis, and even cancer. Inflammation is the body's attempt to remove damaged cells, irritants, pathogens, and harmful stimuli. Swelling, redness, and heat are signs of an acute inflammatory response. Chronic inflammation results from repeated acute inflammation. For instance, if you are constantly stressed, your immune system and stress hormones are always being called on to come to the rescue. Eventually, your immune system wears down, and you "catch" a cold or an infection. If the stress continues, you "catch" more frequent colds and infections until an organ or an organ system in your body becomes too weak to work properly. The end result is a chronic illness.

Autoimmune disease is a chronic illness resulting from an abnormal immune response of either under- or overactivity. The response is abnormal because the immune system attacks substances or tissues normally present in the body. Examples of autoimmune diseases are celiac disease, Guillain-Barré syndrome, IBD, lupus, MS, rheumatoid arthritis, and type 1 diabetes.

Inflammation in the body is widespread, even if it seems to originate from one specific area. People with arthritis have joints that are swollen and hurt. However, they also have inflammation in the arteries, brain, and gums. That's why, once you have one chronic condition, the risk for developing others increases significantly. For example, diabetics are at higher risk for heart and kidney disease.

Persistent inflammation in the brain destroys neurons, increasing vulnerability to memory loss and movement disorders. Immune scavenger cells view toxic beta-amyloid proteins that are present in all brains as "foreign invaders" and launch fierce attacks to remove them. In the process, the scavenger cells overreach and inadvertently destroy millions of healthy brain cells that are essential for memory, thinking, and movement.

Stress, allergens, gum disease, lack of exercise, and toxins in the environment are the main causes of nondietary inflammation. Researchers found that chronic stress alters the effectiveness of cortisol, the stress hormone, to regulate the inflammatory response because it decreases the body's sensitivity to the hormone. This is why chronic stress leads to increasing levels of inflammation if left unchecked.

Exposure to allergens can also cause an immune response of sneezing, coughing, headaches, itching, and breathing problems. All these symptoms are inflammatory responses.

Gum disease consists of swollen gums, an inflammatory response to bacterial growth. If left untreated, bacteria can spread elsewhere in the body and cause problems. People with gum disease have an increased risk of heart disease and cognitive impairment.[1, 2]

As mentioned in Appendix C, exercise has been shown to reduce inflammatory markers in studies. This is likely due to increased energy, better mood and sleep, lower stress levels, and elimination of toxins through sweating. Although not as common as lack of exercise, excessive exercise that doesn't allow time for muscles to repair or the body to get proper rest can actually increase inflammation. For example, weight lifting performed every day on the same muscle groups can damage muscles and increase risk of injury, both inflammatory conditions. Running 50 miles a week to train for marathons can cause adrenal fatigue and joint problems, both signs of chronic inflammation throughout the body.

The main causes of dietary inflammation include food allergens, a diet poor in omega-3 fatty acids and whole-food antioxidants (fruits, vegetables, nuts, and whole grains), and a diet rich in vegetable oils and trans fats, sugar, CAFO-raised meat, dairy products, artificial ingredients, and refined grains.

Foods we are allergic to can cause inflammation throughout the body. The allergy does not need to be severe. A stuffy nose or headache can be caused by a food allergy. Foods that commonly cause allergic reactions are dairy, eggs, peanuts, seafood, soy, tree nuts, and wheat.

The blood test called C-reactive protein (CRP) measures inflammatory agents in the body. Several studies have shown that high blood concentrations of inflammation markers, such as CRP, are associated with a higher risk of dementia and memory impairment. In one large 20-year study, people with the highest CRP levels, as compared to those with the lowest, were more likely to develop cognitive impairment.[3]

Other tests helpful in measuring inflammatory agents are lipid panel, food-allergy profile, and fasting blood glucose. The lipid-panel test measures levels of inflammatory and anti-inflammatory fats. A food-allergy profile identifies food allergens. Avoiding food allergens will reduce inflammation throughout the body.

A fasting blood-glucose test indicates whether blood-sugar levels are normal, high normal, high (prediabetic), or very high (diabetic). Anything but normal means the body has an inflammatory condition. Inflammation can raise blood-sugar levels, and high blood sugar can cause more inflammation—it becomes a vicious cycle. Reducing inflammation naturally is a better option than taking insulin shots.

Below is a list of natural ways to prevent heart disease and other chronic inflammatory conditions.

1. **Exercise regularly.**
   Exercise strengthens the heart, lowers blood pressure, improves mood, keeps weight down, and helps sleep.
2. **Get good-quality sleep.**
   Poor sleep is correlated to increase in heart disease. Review NR7.
3. **Eat a heart-healthy diet.**
   Follow the recommendations in the *Foods Choices* section.

4. **Avoid cigarettes and cigarette smoke.**

   Smoking increases inflammatory responses in the body, therefore increasing risk of many chronic diseases, including coronary heart disease and cancer.

5. **Reduce chronic stress and depression.**

   Chronic stress and depression are associated with higher levels of inflammation and heart disease. Work on changing what you are not happy with in your life. Review NR6.

6. **Maintain good oral hygiene.**

   Floss, brush, and get regular dental cleaning. Take care of any gum problems. Gingivitis and periodontal disease increase risk of heart disease.

7. **Take heart-healthy supplements.**

   Many antioxidants are great for reducing inflammation, including alpha-lipoic acid, CoQ10, curcumin, and quercetin. Magnesium is also critical for heart health. CoQ10 is especially important if you are still taking statins. Quercetin is a flavonoid found in fruits and vegetables that works like an antihistamine and an anti-inflammatory. In addition to reducing tremors by relaxing the nervous system, magnesium regulates heart rhythm and aids in reducing high blood pressure. If you are taking a CCB, let your doctor know before taking magnesium.

8. **Consume fish or take omega-3 supplements.**

   Consume small, wild-caught fish twice a week and/or take an omega-3 EFA supplement daily.

APPENDIX E

Summary of Supplements

Choosing which supplements to buy can be a daunting task. Purchasing from companies that have the GMP (good manufacturing practices) certification, NSF international mark, or US Pharmacopeial (USP) seal of approval on the label can help narrow the search. Supplements with the GMP certification or NSF international mark promise the good manufacturing practices of quality control, cleanliness, identity and potency of ingredients, and testing of final products for potency, purity, and bioavailability.

The Dietary Supplement Validation Program (DSVP) tests products that supplement companies submit to it, followed by inspections of manufacturing facilities to ensure that they meet USP requirements. To ensure that they continue to meet USP standards over time, the DSVP also conducts random aftermarket tests. A committee of stakeholders from industry, government, and consumer groups establish the standards, which include those for identity, potency, purity, bioavailability, and good manufacturing practices.

When it comes to nutritional supplements, you usually get what you pay for in quality and potency with few exceptions. An inexpensive multivitamin with minerals (MVM) usually doesn't contain optimal amounts of beta-carotene, the B vitamins, and vitamin C. Cheaper brands like Centrum and One-A-Day barely contain the RDA, enough to keep you alive, but not enough for optimum health. Plus, both of these brands contain a long list of preservatives and artificial ingredients.

Some of the most expensive supplements are CDP-choline and the powerful antioxidants ALA, astaxanthin, CoQ10, and curcumin. If you can't afford CDP-choline, you can try choline, which costs significantly less. The more fruits and vegetables you consume, the fewer antioxidant supplements your body requires. For Tremor, it's important to take anti-oxidant supplements; however, they are not a substitute for healthy foods. It is more important to eat whole foods than to take supplements if you can't afford both.

If you take medications regularly, make sure you replace any nutrients that the medications deplete. Antidepressants and tranquilizers deplete CoQ10 and riboflavin; cholesterol-lowering drugs deplete CoQ10; ibuprofen depletes folic acid, potassium, and vitamin C; ACE inhibitors deplete zinc, beta-blockers deplete CoQ10 and melatonin, and drugs that regulate blood sugar deplete the B vitamins and CoQ10. Do your own research or ask your pharmacist if the drug you are on depletes any nutrients. Work with your doctor to change the prescription and add back the nutrients that the drug has depleted (or is depleting, if you must continue taking it).

Below is a list of nutritional supplements mentioned throughout this book. You can save money by purchasing combination supplements. Some MVM brands, like Life Extension, contain optimal amounts per serving of vitamins A, B, C, D, and E, ALA, selenium, and zinc. Recommended brands are based on my research and/or experience with them. Any changes in recommendations can be found on my website. See Resources.

Multivitamin with minerals (MVM)

Main benefits: See separate components (vitamins A, B, C, D, and E, magnesium, and zinc) of an MVM below.

Deficiency signs: See separate components of an MVM below.

Optimal dosage: An optimal MVM should contain a minimum of several vitamins and minerals, including 5,000 IU of vitamin A with at least 50 percent in the form of beta-carotene; 25 mg of all the B vitamins except for biotin, folate, and B12, which should have at least 300 mcg, 400 mcg, and 200 mcg, respectively; 500 mg of vitamin C; 1,000 IU of vitamin D; 100 IU of vitamin E in the form of d-alpha tocopherol; 15 mg of zinc; and 200 mcg of selenium. Other minerals usually included in an MVM are calcium, magnesium, copper, manganese, and sometimes chromium or iron. The maximum copper in an MVM should be no more than two mg per daily serving. Only menstruating women or those with a known iron deficiency should take iron. Chromium helps stabilize blood sugar.

Recommended brands:

- Life Extension Two-Per-Day Capsules: supplies 50 mg of B-complex vitamins, 500 mg of vitamin C, 2,000 IU of vitamin D, and 100 IU of vitamin E, plus 25 mg of ALA, 200 mcg of chromium, 200 mcg of selenium, and 30 mg of zinc.
- Alive! Max3 tablets: supplies 25 mg of B-complex vitamins, 1,000 mg of vitamin C, 1,000 IU of vitamin D, and 200 IU of vitamin E, plus 250 mcg of chromium, 200 mcg of selenium, 15 mg of zinc, plus resveratrol, CoQ10, digestive enzymes, and more. Alive! Max3 does not, however, have the preferred forms of folate and vitamin B12.

Vitamin A (NR15)

Main benefits: Powerful antioxidant. Fights free radicals, boosts the immune system, protects night vision, promotes healthy skin, and prevents infections and cancer.

Deficiency signs: Acne, dandruff, diarrhea, frequent colds or infections, and poor night vision.

Best form: Beta-carotene and retinol, with at least 50 percent in the form of beta-carotene.

Optimal dosage: 5,000 to 10,000 IU per day. Sufficient amounts are found in a quality MVM. Additional vitamin A is not needed unless there is a known deficiency.

B complex (NR16)

Main benefits: Supports brain function, healthy skin, nerves, hormone production, energy, fat metabolism, memory, protein digestion, red-cell formation, stress reduction, and healthy hair, nails, and eyes.

Balances blood sugar and aids in use of essential fats. Vitamin B6 is a natural diuretic.

Deficiency signs: Acne, anxiety, bleeding gums, cataracts, constipation, cracked lips, depression, diarrhea, eczema, fatigue, graying hair, headaches, insomnia, irritability, muscle cramps, sore muscles, pale skin, poor concentration, poor hair condition, poor memory, rapid heartbeat, sore tongue, split nails, tremors, and water retention.

Optimal dosage: B-25 or B-50 complex. Each supplement should contain equal amounts (25 or 50 mg) of thiamine, riboflavin, niacinamide, pantothenic acid, and B6, in addition to 50 to 100 mcg of biotin and B12 (methylcobalamin) and 400 to 800 mcg of folate (5-methyl-THF). PABA, choline, and inositol should also be included in a B-complex supplement. Those with memory problems should consider a higher dose and B12 injections.

Cautions: B-complex vitamins are natural diuretics. Taking them with diuretic drugs (water pills) could cause symptoms of dehydration. Niacinamide is preferred to niacin. Niacin can cause skin flushing in some people.

Recommended brands:
- Doctor's Best Fully Active B Complex
- Jarrow Formulas B-Right Complex
- Life Extension Bioactive Complete B Complex

Vitamin C (NR15)

Main benefits: Prevents cell damage, fights free radicals, supports immune function, reduces symptoms of colds, allergies, and stress, improves health of blood vessels, prevents skin wrinkling, detoxifies pollutants, helps make antistress hormones, and turns food into energy.

Deficiency signs: Bleeding gums, dry skin and hair, excessive bruising, frequent colds or infections, joint pain, and low energy.

Best forms: Made from non-GMO ascorbic acid or whole-food, with bioflavonoids.

Optimal dosage: 500 mg per day. Take every four hours during a cold or when feeling run down. Cut back if stools become soft or runny, an indication of more vitamin C than your body can use. Don't worry. Vitamin C has not been found to be toxic at any dosage.

Recommended brands:
- Nutrigold Vitamin C
- Source Naturals Non-GMO C-1000
- Viva Labs Vitamin C
- Pure Synergy Pure Radiance C (capsules or powder)

Vitamin D (NR10)

Main benefits: Promotes absorption of calcium and bone health, boosts immune function, reduces inflammation, supports muscle and nerve function, improves mood, prevents some forms of cancer, and much more.

Deficiency signs: Tooth decay, joint pain and stiffness, muscle cramps, and hair loss.

Best form: Vitamin D3 (cholecalciferol).

Optimal dosage: 1,000 to 2,000 IU per day when combined with the dosage in an MVM. Those who test low or deficient in vitamin D need 5,000 IU or more until blood-serum levels are back to normal.

Caution: Taking high levels of vitamin D2 can result in toxicity symptoms.

Recommended brands:
- Nordic Naturals Vitamin D3
- Doctor's Best Vitamin D3
- Now Foods Vitamin D3
- RealDose Essentials Vegan Vitamin D
- Nordic Naturals Vitamin D3 Vegan
- Garden of Life Mykind Organics 2000 IU Vegan D3 Chewable

Vitamin E (NR15)

Main benefits: Powerful antioxidant. Helps improve wound healing and prevent atherosclerosis, blood clots, cancer, infertility, and thrombosis.

Deficiency signs: Slow wound healing, bruising, infertility, loss of muscle tone, low sex drive, and varicose veins.

Best forms: Mixed tocopherols and tocotrienols or d-alpha tocopherol. Avoid dl-alpha-tocopherol, the synthetic form.

Optimal dosage: 50 to 200 IU a day when combined with the dosage in an MVM. For conditions other than ET, see an alternative healthcare practitioner for proper dosage.

Caution: Vitamin E naturally thins the blood. Taking it with blood-thinning medications can increase risk of bleeding.

Vitamin K (NR10)

Main benefits: Promotes proper blood clotting and helps prevent athero-sclerosis by making sure calcium is transferred to bones instead of calcifying in arteries.

Deficiency signs: Easy bleeding, varicose veins, tooth decay, and bone weakness.

Best forms: K2 and MK-7.

Optimal dosage: 30 to 90 mcg per day. Vitamin K supplementation is important when taking calcium supplements.

Caution: Vitamin K naturally thins the blood. Taking it with blood-thinning medications can increase risk of bleeding.

Recommended brands:
- Doctor's Best Natural Vitamin K2
- Life Extension Low-Dose Vitamin K2
- Now Foods MK-7

Choline (NR17)

Main benefits: Supports brain and nerve health, improves cognitive func-tion, reduces inflammation, and helps break down fat in the liver.

Deficiency signs: Atherosclerosis, dementia, high blood pressure, and nerve degeneration.

Best forms: CDP-choline (citicoline) or choline.

Optimal dosage: 250 to 400 mg per day.

Recommended brands:

- Jarrow Formulas CDP Choline
- Life Extension Cognizon CDP-Choline Caps
- Now Foods Choline & Inositol

Omega-3 EFAs (NR3 and Appendix D)

Main benefits: Supports brain and nervous system function, lowers inflammation, improves mood, reduces hyperactivity, helps in preventing memory loss and dementia, helps balance hormones, and reduces insulin resistance.

Deficiency signs: Poor memory and learning difficulties, dry skin and eczema, depression, excessive thirst and sweating, and inflammatory conditions such as arthritis and diabetes.

Best forms: Marine microalgae, fish oil, cod liver oil, and flaxseed oil or meal. For fish oils, look for brands free of PCBs. Flaxseed oil should be cold pressed and unrefined. Flaxseed meal should be kept in the refrigerator and used by the expiration date. Regardless of expiration date, it's rancid if it smells or tastes fishy.

Optimal dosage: 1,000 mg of combined EPA and DHA or 2,000 mg of flaxseed oil per day. Take with food that contains some fat for better absorption.

Recommended brands:

- Nordic Naturals Algae Omega
- Deva Vegan Omega-3 (algae)
- Nordic Naturals Omega-3 (fish)
- Now Foods Omega-3 (fish)
- Carlson Cod Liver Oil (also contains vitamin D3)
- Deva Vegan Flaxseed Oil
- Barlean's Flax Oil

- Now Foods Flax Oil
- Bob's Red Mill Flaxseed Meal

Magnesium (NR18 and Appendix D)

Main benefits: Calms nerves, promotes normal blood pressure, keeps bones strong, helps maintain a healthy heart rhythm, and maintains proper muscle function.

Deficiency signs: Confusion, constipation, depression, hyperactivity, kidney stones, lack of appetite, muscle tremors or spasms, muscle weakness, high blood pressure, insomnia, irregular heartbeat, and nervousness.

Best forms: Chloride, citrate, glycinate, malate, orotate, taurate, and L-threonate.

Optimal dosage: For tremors, take 600 to 1,200 mg depending on severity of symptoms and other signs of a magnesium deficiency. When taking more than 600 mg, split the dose between morning and evening or divide it evenly with meals.

Caution: Too much of certain forms of magnesium may cause loose stools. Cut back a little or change to a different form if that happens.

Recommended brands:
- Doctor's Best High Absorption Magnesium
- Life Extension Magnesium Citrate
- Now Foods Magnesium Citrate Pure Powder

Zinc (NR14)

Main benefits: Increases energy, promotes a healthy nervous system and brain, aids in coping with stress, controls hormones, removes toxins, heals wounds, supports reproductive health, and is important for learning and memory.

Deficiency signs: Acne, diarrhea, frequent infections, loss of appetite, reduced sense of smell, and white spots on nails.

Best forms: Zinc acetate, citrate, gluconate, sulfate, and picolinate.

Optimal dosage: 15 to 30 mg when combined with the dosage in an MVM.

Alpha–lipoic acid (NR15 and Appendix D)

Main benefits: Reduces damage to cells, aids insulin in lowering blood sugar, and reduces and prevents inflammation.

Deficiency signs: Inflammatory conditions: allergies, bags under eyes, bloating, erectile dysfunction, gum disease, high blood sugar, joint pain, excessive weight, and skin problems (acne, puffiness, redness, and rashes).

Optimal dosage: 30 to 100 mg per day. Additional amounts are needed for treating specific inflammatory conditions—see an alternative healthcare practitioner for proper dosage.

Caution: ALA naturally lowers blood sugar; taking it with diabetic drugs, which do the same, raises the risk of hypoglycemia.

Recommended brands:
- Doctor's Best Alpha-Lipoic Acid
- Jarrow Formulas Alpha Lipoic Acid
- Now Foods Alpha Lipoic Acid
- Source Naturals Alpha Lipoic Acid

Astaxanthin (NR15)

Main benefits: Powerful antioxidant and anti-inflammatory. Protects skin from sun damage by acting as a natural sunscreen. Protects eyes from diabetic retinopathy and macular degeneration. May protect against arthritis, cancer, chronic fatigue, gastric ulcers, heart disease, kidney damage from diabetes, and neurodegeneration.

Deficiency signs: Any chronic inflammatory condition, vision problems, and sunburn.

Best form: Natural variety from marine algae.

Optimal dosage: 4 to 12 mg per day. Those with arthritis, diabetes, or vision problems should take 12 mg daily or 4 mg, three times per day.

Recommended brands:
- Health Ranger's Hawaiian Astaxanthin
- Nutrex BioAstin Hawaiian Astaxanthin
- Viva Labs Astaxanthin
- Deva Vegan Astaxanthin

Coenzyme Q10 (NR15 and Appendix D)

Main benefits: Powerful antioxidant that protects cells from damage, helps prevent heart and gum disease, and boosts immune function.

Deficiency signs: Chronic pain, weak immune function, heart disease, and fatigue.

Best forms: Ubiquinol and ubiquinone.

Optimal dosage: 30 to 50 mg per day. Those with gum disease or HBP should take 50 mg to 100 mg, twice daily. Those with congestive heart failure, heart disease, chronic fatigue, fibromyalgia, or who are taking statins should take 100 to 150 mg, twice daily.

Recommended brands:
- Now Foods CoQ10 (50 and 100 mg softgels)
- Now Foods CoQ10 Vcaps (30, 60, 100, and 150 mg)
- Doctor's Best High Absorption CoQ10 (100 mg softgels)
- Doctor's Best High Absorption CoQ10 Veggie Caps (100 mg)
- Viva Labs CoQ10 (100 mg softgels)

Curcumin (NR15 and Appendix D)

Main benefits: Powerful antioxidant and anti-inflammatory. Protects neurons from free-radical damage and helps prevent cancer and heart disease.

Best form: Curcumin C3 or turmeric capsules with minimum 95 percent curcuminoids and piperine (black pepper extract). Piperine makes curcumin more absorbable.

Optimal dosage: 300 to 500 mg per day. Take every four hours for headaches and two to three times per day for arthritis.

Cautions: Turmeric helps prevent gallstones by promoting gallbladder emptying, but for those with existing gallstones, it could increase the risk of symptoms. In addition, turmeric naturally thins blood, so taking it with blood-thinning medications can increase risk of bleeding.

Recommended brands:

- Pure Sun Naturals Turmeric Curcumin (500 mg vegetarian capsules)
- Viva Labs Turmeric Curcumin C³ Complex (500 mg vegetarian capsules)
- Incredipure Turmeric Curcumin (750 mg vegetarian capsules)

Garlic (NR14 and Appendix B)

Main benefits: Antibacterial, antifungal, anticoagulant, antioxidant, and antiviral properties. Helps fight and prevent stomach ulcers, infections (fungal, staphylococcus, MRSA, and others), colds, and viruses (including the flu). Thins blood and may help lower blood pressure.

Best forms: Organic garlic in capsules or softgels.

Optimal dosage: Take 400 to 600 mg once a day for heart health and to prevent illness. Take two to three a day to help get rid of an infection or cold. For lowering blood pressure or thinning blood, see a healthcare practitioner for proper dosage.

Caution: Garlic naturally thins the blood. Taking it with blood-thinning medications can increase risk of bleeding.

Recommended brand:

- Kyolic Aged Garlic Extract. Kyolic is odorless and burpless.

Quercetin (Appendix D)

Main benefits: Antihistamine, anti-inflammatory, and antioxidant properties. Quercetin helps reduce allergy symptoms by blocking histamines, and it helps prevent heart disease by inhibiting buildup of plaque in arteries.

Deficiency signs: Allergy symptoms and dark circles under eyes.

Best form: Quercetin with bromelain for easier absorption.

Optimal dosage: For cardiovascular health, take 400 mg per day. For heart disease and allergy symptoms during allergy season, take two a day—one in the morning and one in the evening. Take 20 minutes before meals.

Recommended brand:

- Amazing Nutrition Quercetin Bromelain

Amino acids GABA, glutamine, glycine, and theanine (NR19)

Main benefits: Relieve anxiety, improve sleep, promote mental and physical calm, and may reduce tremors in ET.

Deficiency signs: Anxiety, chronic pain, depression, hyperactivity, and insomnia.

Best form: Best when used in combination with other calming herbs and supplements.

Optimal dosage: Supplement that contains at least 200 mg of GABA in combination with other amino acids and calming herbs. Some people need as much as 500 mg for best results. Any dose over 500 mg should be monitored by a healthcare practitioner.

Cautions: These supplements cause drowsiness. They are best taken at bedtime and never before driving or operating machinery. In addition, taking them with alcohol or the drugs alprazolam, benzodiazepines, and other CNS sedatives can cause extreme drowsiness.

Recommended brands:

- Now Foods True Calm (contains valerian, GABA, glycine, and taurine)
- Source Naturals GABA Calm (contains GABA, N-acetyl L-tyrosine, glycine, and taurine)

Relaxing herbs (NR20)

Main benefits: Calms the nervous system—reduces anxiety, stress, shaking, headaches, and other nerve-related symptoms.

Recommended herbs: Chamomile, hops, passionflower, skullcap, and valerian

Optimal dosage: Take as directed on package.

Cautions: These supplements cause drowsiness. They are best taken at bedtime and never before driving or operating machinery. In addition, taking them with alcohol or the drugs alprazolam, benzodiazepines, and other CNS sedatives can cause extreme drowsiness.

Recommended brands:
- Now Foods Sleep (contains GABA, valerian, passionflower, and hops)
- Now Foods True Calm (contains valerian, GABA, glycine, and taurine)
- The Vitamin Shoppe Snooze Right (contains chamomile, passionflower, hops, skullcap, valerian, inositol, and L-taurine)

Melatonin (NR6, NR7)

Main benefits: Antioxidant and sleep aid.

Deficiency signs: Insomnia, restless sleep, and fatigue.

Optimal dosage: Take 0.3 mg (300 mcg) to 1 mg, 30 to 60 minutes before bedtime. Start with 0.3 mg and slowly increase dose for best sleep.

Cautions: Too much melatonin can cause dizziness, headaches, nausea, or irritability.

5-HTP (NR6, NR7)

Main benefits: Contains tryptophan which is converted to serotonin in the body. Serotonin is a natural antidepressant, appetite suppressant, and sleep aid.

Deficiency signs: Constipation, depression, insomnia, and mood disorders.

Best form: 5-hydroxytryptophan.

Optimal dosage: For treating insomnia, start with 100 mg of 5-HTP, taken before bedtime. It can take up to three months to work. If 100 mg doesn't improve sleep, increase dose to 200 mg. For treating anxiety and depression, start with 50 mg of 5-HTP, three times per day, 30 minutes before meals. Increase dose to 75 or 100 mg if 50 mg doesn't help alleviate depression after three months. Seek advice from a healthcare practitioner for higher doses.

Caution: Never take 5-HTP with antidepressants, L-tryptophan, or any other medications or supplements that increase serotonin levels without a doctor's approval and monitoring.

Digestive enzymes (Appendix A)

Main benefit: Aids in the breakdown of food to ensure proper digestion of nutrients.

Deficiency signs: Allergies, chronic fatigue, gum disease, obesity, pancreatitis, skin problems, ulcers, and too many other symptoms to list.

Best forms: Plant-based enzymes derived from aspergillus. Animal-based versions may work better for those who've had pancreatitis or gallstones. Each supplement should contain protease for digesting proteins, amylase for digesting carbohydrates, lipase to break down fats, and lactase for those who are lactose intolerant. Bromelain from pineapple can be used alone or with other enzymes by those who have allergies, arthritis, or other inflammatory conditions.

Optimal dosage: Take as directed on package.

Recommended brands:
- Now Foods Optimal Digestive System
- Zenwise Advanced Digestive Enzymes (with probiotics)

Probiotics (Appendix A)

Main benefit: Increase beneficial bacteria in the gut.

Deficiency signs: Abdominal pain and cramping, bad breath, bloating, constipation, diarrhea, frequent infections, fatigue, gas, and neurological problems.

Best forms: The most effective probiotic supplement should include lactobacillus acidophilus and bifidobacteria bifidum in addition to any combination of lactobacillus salivarius, lactobacillus bulgaricus, lactobacillus casei, bifidobacteria infantis, bifidobacteria brevis, bifidobacteria longum, bacillus coagulans, and streptococcus thermophilus.

Optimal dosage: Take as directed on package.

Recommended brands:

- Garden of Life Primal Defense
- Now Foods Probiotic-10
- Renew Life Ultimate Flora
- Zenwise Advanced Digestive Enzymes (with probiotics)

Chlorella (NR13)

Main benefits: Eliminates toxins including aluminum and mercury, and helps prevent toxic accumulation in the CNS.

Best form: Tablets, capsules, or powder.

Optimal dosage: 1,000 to 2,000 mg (1 to 2 grams) per day for maintenance. For detoxing metals, start with 1,000 mg and build to 5,000 mg per day. Take with meals, spread evenly.

Recommended brand:

- Clean Chlorella by Health Ranger Select. The company tests their products rigorously for radiation and other contaminants. Tablets are small and easy to swallow. Five tablets equal 1 gram. Instead of worrying how to divide 5, 10, or 25 tablets by three meals, take 2 to 3 tablets with each meal for maintenance and 5 to 8 with each meal for detoxing metals.

Progesterone (NR8)

Main benefits: Balances hormones and blood sugar, increases metabolism, reduces visceral fat, promotes normal sleep, stimulates bone production, and alleviates anxiety and depression. Natural diuretic. May be beneficial for treating menopausal hot flashes and premenstrual syndrome (PMS).

Signs of progesterone imbalance: Anxiety, breast tenderness, cravings, depression, fatigue, headaches, heavy periods, irritability, low libido, restless sleep, and weight gain.

Best form: Natural, or bioidentical, transdermal creams. Avoid synthetic progesterone (progestin).

Optimal dosage: Use as directed on package or by a healthcare practitioner.

Caution: Do not take long term without having lab tests performed to determine proper dosage.

Recommended brands:
- Emerita Pro-Gest Cream
- Life-Flo Progesta-Care
- Now Foods Progesterone Cream

RESOURCES

Part I: Overview

www.essentialtremor.org

This is the website for the International Essential Tremor Foundation (IETF). The IETF funds research to find the cause of ET that leads to treatments and a cure, increases awareness, and provides educational materials, tools, and support for healthcare providers, the public, and those affected by ET. The website includes tips for everyone living with ET.

www.tremoraction.org

Tremor Action Network (TAN) is a nonprofit founded in 2003 by people diagnosed with essential tremor, cervical dystonia, and Parkinson's disease. TAN is dedicated to providing boutique services that include one-on-one support and guidance to patients, family members, and caregivers.

Part II: Conventional Treatments

www.drugs.com

A comprehensive source of information on more than 24,000 prescription drugs, over-the-counter medicines, and natural products.

www.clinicaltrials.gov

A registry and results database of publicly and privately supported clinical studies of human participants conducted around the world. To find all studies on ET, both completed and in progress, type "Essential Tremor" in the *Search for Studies* search box.

Part III: Natural Remedies
NR1. Fear Frankenfoods

Elisabeth Hasselbeck, *The G-Free Diet: A Gluten-Free Survival Guide* (New York: Hachette Book Group, 2009)

David Perlmutter, *Grain Brain: The Surprising Truth about Wheat, Carbs, and Sugar—Your Brain's Silent Killer* (New York: Hachette Book Group, 2013)

NR2. Eliminate Excitotoxins
Russell L. Blaylock, *Excitotoxins: The Taste That Kills* (Santa Fe: Health Press, 1997)

Janet Starr Hull, *Sweet Poison: How the World's Most Popular Artificial Sweetener Is Killing Us—My Story* (Far Hills: New Horizon Press, 2001)

NR3. Opt for Brain-Healthy Fats
Jonny Bowden and Stephen Sinatra, *The Great Cholesterol Myth: Why Lowering Your Cholesterol Won't Prevent Heart Disease and the Statin-Free Plan That Will* (Beverly: Fair Winds Press, 2012)

Jack Challem, *The Inflammation Syndrome: Your Nutrition Plan for Great Health, Weight Loss, and Pain-Free Living* (Hoboken, NJ: John Wiley & Sons, 2010)

Anthony Colpo, *The Great Cholesterol Con* (Lulu.com, 2012)

Bruce Fife, *The Coconut Oil Miracle* (New York: Penguin Group, 2013)

Barbara H. Roberts, *The Truth About Statins: Risks and Alternatives to Cholesterol-Lowering Drugs* (New York: Gallery Books, 2012)

NR6. Reduce Stress
Joe Dominquez and Vicki Robin, *Your Money or Your Life: 9 Steps to Transforming Your Relationship with Money and Achieving Financial Independence* (New York: Penguin Books, 2008)

NR8. Balance Hormones
Thierry Hertoghe, *The Hormone Solution: Stay Younger Longer with Natural Hormone and Nutrition Therapies* (New York: Three Rivers Press, 2002)

John R. Lee, *What Your Doctor May Not Tell You about Menopause (TM): The Breakthrough Book on Natural Hormone Balance* (New York: Time Warner Book Group, 2004)

NR9. Avoid Tremor-Inducing Drugs

James F. Balch, *Prescription for Drug Alternatives: All-Natural Options for Better Health without the Side Effects* (Hoboken, NJ: John Wiley & Sons, 2008)

Elson M. Haas, *The Detox Diet: The Definitive Guide for Lifelong Vitality with Recipes, Menus, and Detox Plans* (New York: Ten Speed Press, 2012)

www.swisswater.com
The Swiss Water Decaffeinated Coffee Company specializes in making decaffeinated coffee without chemicals.

NR11. Electromagnetic Fields

Martin Blank, *Overpowered: The Dangers of Electromagnetic Radiation (EMF) and What You Can Do about It* (New York: Seven Stories Press, 2014)

Ann Louise Gittleman, *Zapped: Why Your Cell Phone Shouldn't Be Your Alarm Clock and 1,268 Ways to Outsmart the Hazards of Electronic Pollution* (New York: HarperCollins, 2010)

Katie Singer, *An Electronic Silent Spring: Facing the Dangers and Creating Safe Limits* (Great Barrington: Portal Books, 2014)

www.electricsense.com
Developed by Lloyd Burrell who cured himself of EHS, this website contains information on the dangers of cell phones, cordless phones, smart meters, and other wireless technology. It also has information on how to buy an EMF meter to evaluate your risk, and steps you can take to protect yourself from radiation poisoning in your home and environment.

www.emfwise.com
Based on approximately seven years of follow-up on EMF news and literature, this site, based in the United States, aims to provide a rational and
scientific perspective on electromagnetic fields as well as precautionary
and prevention measures to minimize health risks.

https://takebackyourpower.net
Take Back Your Power is an award-winning documentary film directed
and produced by Josh del Sol that investigates so-called "smart" utility
meters, uncovering shocking evidence of the in-home privacy invasions,
increased utility bills, health and environmental harm, fires, and hacking
vulnerability—and lights the path toward solutions. The website also contains a step-by-step action guide on how to "take back your power" and
recommended books on the dangers of smart meters and EMFs.

NR12. Household Chemicals
www.localharvest.org
Lists local farms or farmers that participate in community-supported agriculture (CSA) and has information on local farmers' markets.

NR14. Vaccinations
www.cdc.gov/vaccines/pubs/pinkbook/downloads/appendices/B/excipi-
ent-table-2.pdf
Lists ingredients in vaccines by vaccine and manufacturer.

drjeandoddspethealthresource.tumblr.com
Provides information on vaccine protocols, thyroid issues, and nutrition
for pets.

NR18. Magnesium
Carolyn Dean, *The Magnesium Miracle* (New York: Ballantine Books, 2007)

NR23. Homeopathy

Asa Hershoff, *Homeopathic Remedies: A Quick and Easy Guide to Common Disorders and Their Homeopathic Remedies* (New York: Avery Publishing, 2000)

Ambika Wauters, *The Homeopathy Bible: The Definitive Guide to Remedies* (New York: Sterling Publishing, 2007)

Nutritional Supplements

www.iherb.com

The company sells nutritional supplements, herbs, bath and beauty products, and more. Prices are competitive. They offer free shipping with an order of $20 or more, and a discount off subsequent orders, calculated as 10 percent of your current order, if purchased within 60 days.

www.lifeextension.com

Quality nutritional supplements, herbs, hormones, and skin care. Blood tests are also available at reasonable prices. Some Life Extension supplements can also be purchased at iHerb.com and Amazon.com.

www.healthfitnesscafe.blogspot.com

The author's website. It contains up-to-date news and information on health-related topics. The HFC Store has supplements recommended for ET and other health conditions.

ENDNOTES

1. Tremors Defined

1. Eliezer Sternberg et al., "Postural and Intention Tremors: A Detailed Clinical Study of Essential Tremor vs. Parkinson's Disease," National Center for Biotechnology Information, accessed April 4, 2016, http://www.ncbi.nlm.nih.gov/pmc/articles/PMC3650675/.

2. "What Causes Parkinson's?" Parkinson's Disease Foundation, accessed April 4, 2014, http://www.pdf.org/en/causes.

3. "Tremor Fact Sheet," National Institute of Neurological Disorders and Stroke," accessed April 4, 2014, http://www.ninds.nih.gov/disorders/tremor/detail_tremor.htm.

4. Ibid.

5. Ibid.

6. "Dystonias Fact Sheet," National Institute of Neurological Disorders and Stroke," accessed April 4, 2014, http://www.ninds.nih.gov/disorders/dysto-nias/detail_dystonias.htm.

7. "Dystonia: Treatment," Mayo Clinic, accessed April 5, 2016, http://www.mayoclinic.org/diseases-conditions/dystonia/diagnosis-treatment/treatment/txc-20163708.

8. Ibid.

9. J. Eric Ahlskog, "Orthostatic Tremor Significantly Affects Quality of Life," Mayo Clinic News Network, accessed May 4, 2014, http://newsnetwork.mayoclinic.org/discussion/orthostatic-tremor-significantly-affects-quality-of-life.

10. Ibid.

11. Ibid.

12. Ibid.

13. Ibid.

14. "Psychogenic Movement," Brain Facts, accessed April 4, 2014, http://www.brainfacts.org/diseases-disorders/diseases-a-to-z-from-ninds/psychogenic-movement/.

15. Ibid.
16. Juan Pablo Romero, Julián Benito-León, and Félix Bermejo-Pareja, "The NEDICES Study: Recent Advances in the Understanding of the Epidemiology of Essential Tremor," National Center for Biotechnology Information, accessed May 4, 2014, http://www.ncbi.nlm.nih.gov/pmc/articles/PMC3570054/.

2. Possible Causes and Risks

1. Carles Vilariño-Güell et al., "LINGO1 and LINGO2 Variants Are Associated with Essential Tremor and Parkinson Disease," National Center for Biotechnology Information, accessed October 4, 2012, http://www.ncbi.nlm.nih.gov/pmc/articles/PMC3930084/.
2. "Researchers Identify Likely Cause of Essential Tremor," News-Medical (blog), December 7, 2011, http://www.news-medical.net/news/20111207/Researchers-identify-likely-cause-of-essential-tremor.aspx.
3. B. Koster et al., "Essential Tremor and Cerebellar Dysfunction: Abnormal Ballistic Movements," Journal of Neurology, Neurosurgery, and Psychiatry 73, no. 4 (2002): 400–05.
4. Allison Gandey, "Heavy Drinking Doubles Risk for Essential Tremor Later in Life," Medscape (blog), April 21, 2009, http://www.medscape.org/viewarticle/701660.
5. Okan Dogu et al., "Elevated Blood Lead Concentrations in Essential Tremor: A Case-Control Study in Mersin, Turkey," Environmental Health Perspectives 115, no. 11 (2007): 1564–68.
6. J. Benito-León et al., "Elderly Onset Essential Tremor and Mild Cognitive Impairment: A Population Based Study (NEDICES)," Journal of Alzheimer's Disease 23, no. 4 (2011): 727–735, accessed October 4, 2012, doi: 10.3233/JAD-2011-101572.
7. Ibid.
8. W. G. Ondo et al., "Hearing Impairment in Essential Tremor," Neurology 61, no. 8 (2003): 1093–97, accessed October 4, 2012, http://www.ncbi.nlm.nih.gov/pubmed/14581670.

9. Elan D. Louis et al., "Frailty in Elderly Persons with Essential Tremor: A Population-Based Study (NEDICES)," *European Journal of Neurology*, 18, no. 10 (2011): 1251–57, accessed October 4, 2012, doi: 10.1111/j.1468-1331.2011.03374.x.
10. Aron S. Buchman et al., "Physical Frailty in Older Persons is Associated with Alzheimer Disease Pathology," *Neurology* 71, no. 7 (2008): 499–504.

3. Symptoms

1. "Essential Tremor (ET)," John Hopkins Medicine, accessed April 9, 2016, http://www.hopkinsmedicine.org/healthlibrary/conditions/nervous_system_disorders/essential_tremor_disorder_134,30/.
2. "Essential Tremor," Medline Plus, accessed May 10, 2016, https://www.nlm.nih.gov/medlineplus/ency/article/000762.htm.
3. "Essential Tremor: Description," Genetics Home Reference, accessed May 10, 2016, https://ghr.nlm.nih.gov/condition/essential-tremor.

4. Diagnosis

1. "Wilson's Disease: Definition," Mayo Clinic, accessed October 4, 2012, http://www.mayoclinic.org/diseases-conditions/wilsons-disease/basics/definition/con-20043499?reDate=09122014.
2. "Essential Tremor: The Family Health Guide," Harvard Health Publications, accessed February 17, 2015, http://www.health.harvard.edu/diseases-and-conditions/essential-tremor-the.

5. Pharmaceutical Drugs

1. "Common Medications," International Essential Tremor Foundation, accessed April 6, 2016, http://www.essentialtremor.org/treatments/medication/.
2. Ibid.

3. W. Ondo et al., "Gabapentin for Essential Tremor: A Multiple-dose, Double-blind, Placebo-controlled Trial," PubMed, accessed April 6, 2014, http://www.ncbi.nlm.nih.gov/pubmed/10928578.
4. "Perampanel Study," International Essential Tremor Foundation," accessed July 14, 2016, http://www.essentialtremor.org/research/research-recruitment/perampanel-study/.

6. Surgery

1. "Deep Brain Stimulation: What You Can Expect," Mayo Clinic, accessed April 10, 2016, http://www.mayoclinic.org/tests-proce-dures/deep-brain-stimulation/details/what-you-can-expect/rec-20156715.
2. "Deep Brain Stimulation: Risks," Mayo Clinic, accessed April 10, 2016, http://www.mayoclinic.org/tests-procedures/deep-brain-stimulation/details/risks/cmc-20156104.
3. "Deep Brain Stimulation," Medline Plus, accessed April 14, 2016, https://www.nlm.nih.gov/medlineplus/ency/article/007453.htm.
4. "Essential Tremor: Surgical Options," International Essential Tremor Foundation, accessed April 10, 2014, http://www.essentialtremor.org/wp-content/uploads/2013/07/Surgical-Options-050913.pdf.
5. "What is Gamma Knife?" Gamma Knife for Tremor, accessed April 14, 2016, http://www.gammaknifefortremor.com/?page_id=2930.
6. American Society for Radiation Oncology, "Stereotactic Radiosurgery as Effective in Eliminating Parkinson's Disease Tremors as Other Treatments but Less Invasive," Science Daily (blog), November 2, 2009, www.science-daily.com/releases/2009/11/091102121504.htm.
7. "Essential Tremor and Stereotactic Thalamotomy," WebMD, accessed April 16, 2016, http://www.webmd.com/brain/essential-tremor-stereotactic-thalamotomy.
8. Ibid.
9. Tracey Denninger, "Essential Tremor Treatment Shows Promise," Today's Geriatric Medicine (blog), accessed October 6, 2014, http://todaysgeriatricmedicine.com/news/ex_040312.shtml.

10. W. J. Elias et al., "A Pilot Study of Focused Ultrasound Thalamotomy for Essential Tremor," *New England Journal of Medicine* 369, no. 7 (2015): 640–48.

11. Lipsman et al., "MRI-Guided Focused Ultrasound Thalamotomy."

12. "Essential Tremor: Surgical Options," International Essential Tremor Foundation, accessed April 10, 2014, http://www.essentialtremor.org/wp-content/uploads/2013/07/Surgical-Options-050913.pdf.

7. Other Options

1. "Treatment Options: Botulinum Toxin Injections," Essential Tremor, accessed April 18, 2016, http://www.essentialtremor.org/treatments/botox/.

2. Mark Plumb and Peter Bain, *Essential Tremor: The Facts*, (New York: Oxford University Press, 2007), 58.

3. "Treatment Options: Common Medications," Essential Tremor, accessed April 18, 2016, http://www.essentialtremor.org/treatments/medication/.

4. Monique Giroux, MD, "Marijuana and Tremor," Essential Tremor, accessed April 18, 2016, http://essentialtremor.org/wp-content/uploads/2014/05/TremorTalkApril2014FINAL.pdf.

NR1. Fear Frankenfoods

1. Nancy L. Lawson et al., "Genetically Engineered Crops, Glyphosate and the Deterioration of Health in the United States of America," *Journal of Organic Systems* 9, no. 2 (2014): 6–33, http://www.organic-systems.org/journal/92/abstracts/Swanson-et-al.html.

2. Grace Rattue, "Autoimmune Disease Rates Increasing," *Medical News Today* (blog), June 22, 2012, http://www.medicalnewstoday.com/articles/246960.php.

3. Caroline Cassels, "Updated Rates of US Neurological Disorders Show Increased MS, AD Prevalence," *Medscape* (blog), January 29, 2007, http://www.medscape.com/viewarticle/551439.

4. C. Pritchard, A. Mayers, and D. Baldwin, "Changing Patterns of Neurological Mortality in the 10 Major Developed Countries, 1979–2010," *Public Health*, 127, no.4 (2013): 357–68.

5. "Recombinant Bovine Growth Hormone," American Cancer Society, accessed April 29, 2015, http://www.cancer.org/cancer/cancercauses/othercarcinogens/athome/recombinant-bovine-growth-hormone.

6. William J. Cromie, "Growth Factor Raises Cancer Risk," *The Harvard University Gazette* (blog), April 22, 1999, http://news.harvard.edu/gazette/1999/04.22/igf1.story.html.

7. Y. Lurie et al., "Celiac Disease Diagnosed in the Elderly," *Journal of Clinical Gastroenterology* 42, no. 1 (2008): 59–61.

8. Kimberly Wonderly, "Gluten Sensitivity & Parkinson's Disease," *Livestrong* (blog), April 16, 2013, http://www.livestrong.com/article/549400-gluten-sensitivity-parkinsons-disease/.

9. William Davis, *Wheat Belly: Lose the Wheat, Lose the Weight, and Find Your Path Back to Health* (New York: Rodale, 2011), 60–61.

10. Ibid., 9.

11. Stéphanie Debette et al., "Visceral Fat is Associated with Lower Brain Volume in Healthy Middle-Aged Adults," *Annals of Neurology* 68, no. 2 (2010): 136–144.

NR2. Eliminate Excitotoxins

1. Russell L. Blaylock, *Excitotoxins: The Taste That Kills.* (Santa Fe: Health Press, 1997), 191-204.

2. Steven Reinberg, "Study Suggests Brain Damage in 40 Percent of Ex-NFL Players," *US News & World Report*, April 11, 2016, http://health.usnews.com/health-news/articles/2016-04-11/study-suggests-brain-damage-in-40-percent-of-ex-nfl-players.

3. Helen Scholz, "Aspartame," *Side Effects* (blog), February 28, 2011, http://www.sideeffects.com/aspartame.html.

4. Russell L. Blaylock, "Food Additive Excitotoxins and Degenerative Brain Disorders," *Whale.to*, accessed October 8, 2012, http://www.whale.to/a/blaylock5.html.

5. American College of Cardiology, "Too Many Diet Drinks May Spell Heart Trouble for Older Women, Study Suggests," *Science Daily* (blog), March 29, 2014, http://www.sciencedaily.com/releases/2014/03/140329175110.htm.

6. Arthur M. Evangelista, "History of Aspartame," World National Health Organization, accessed October 8, 2012, http://www.wnho.net/history_of_aspartame.htm.

7. Ibid.

8. Ibid.

9. Janet Starr Hull, "Dangers of Aspartame Poisoning," in *Sweet Poison*, accessed October 8, 2012, http://www.sweetpoison.com/aspartame-information.html.

10. Weizmann Institute of Science, "Certain Gut Bacteria May Induce Metabolic Changes Following Exposure to Artificial Sweeteners," *Science Daily* (blog), September 17, 2014, http://www.sciencedaily.com/releases/2014/09/140917131634.htm.

11. Katherine Zeratsky, "Monosodium Glutamate (MSG): Is It Harmful?" Mayo Clinic, accessed June 7, 2010, http://www.mayoclinic.org/healthy-living/nutrition-and-healthy-eating/expert-answers/monosodium-glutamate/faq-20058196.

12. Blaylock, *Excitotoxins*, 255.

13. Ibid., 218.

14. Ibid., 182–83.

15. Blaylock, "Food Additive Excitotoxins," accessed June 7, 2010.

NR3. Opt for Brain-Healthy Fats

1. Anthony Colpo, *The Great Cholesterol Con: Why Everything You've Been Told about Cholesterol, Diet and Heart Disease is Wrong!* (Raleigh: Lulu, 2006), 38.

2. Catherine Paddock, "Experts Question Link between Saturated Fat and Heart Disease," *Medical News Today* (blog), March 18, 2014, http://www.medicalnewstoday.com/articles/274166.php.

3. Patty W. Siri-Tarino, "Meta-Analysis of Prospective Cohort Studies Evaluating the Association of Saturated Fat with Cardiovascular Disease," *American Journal of Clinical Nutrition* 91, no. 3 (2010): 535–46.

4. Chris Masterjohn, "Myth: Eating Cholesterol-Rich Foods Raises Cholesterol Levels," *Cholesterol and Health* (blog), September 20, 2007, http://

www.cholesterol-and-health.com/Cholesterol-Rich-Foods-Raise-Blood-Cholesterol.html.

5. Bruce Fife, *Stop Alzheimer's Now! How to Prevent and Reverse Dementia, Multiple Sclerosis, and Other Neurodegenerative Disorders* (Colorado Springs: Piccadilly Books, 2011), 169.

6. Ibid., 203.

7. Nikolaos Scarmeas and Elan D. Louis, "Mediterranean Diet and Essential Tremor," *Neuroepidemiology*, 29, no. 3–4 (2007): 170–177.

8. Colpo, *Great Cholesterol Con*, 44–45.

9. A. P. Simopoulos, "The Importance of the Ratio of Omega-6/Omega-3 Essential Fatty Acids," *Biomedicine and Pharmacotherapy* 56, no. 8 (2002): 365–79.

10. L. Buydens-Branchey et al., "Associations Between Increases in Plasma n-3 Polyunsaturated Fatty Acids Following Supplementation and Decreases in Anger and Anxiety in Substance Abusers," *Progress in Neuro-Psychopharmacology & Biological Psychiatry* 32, no. 2 (2008): 568–75.

11. G. Fontani et al., "Blood Profiles, Body Fat and Mood State in Healthy Subjects on Different Diets Supplemented with Omega-3 Polyunsaturated Fatty Acids," *European Journal of Clinical Investigation* 35, no. 8 (2005): 499–507.

12. C. T. Chen et al., "Rapid De-Esterification and Loss of Eicosapentaenoic Acid from Rat Brain Phospholipids: An Intracerebroventricular Study," *Journal of Neurochemistry* 116, no. 3 (2011): 363–73.

13. Gwendolyn Barceló-Coblijn et al., "Flaxseed Oil and Fish-Oil Capsule Consumption Alters Human Red Blood Cell n-3 Fatty Acid Composition: A Multiple-Dosing Trial Comparing 2 Sources of n-3 Fatty Acid," *American Journal of Clinical Nutrition* 88, no. 3 (2008): 801–809.

14. Masterjohn, "Myth."

15. A. Saremi et al., "Progression of Vascular Calcification Is Increased with Statin Use in the Veterans Affairs Diabetes Trial (VADT)." *Diabetes Care* 35, no. 11 (2012): 2390–92.

16. Colpo, *Great Cholesterol Con*, 19.

17. Staffan Nilsson et al., "No Connection between the Level of Exposition to Statins in the Population and the Incidence/Mortality of Acute Myocardial Infarction: An Ecological Study Based on Sweden's Municipalities," *Journal of Negative Results in Biomedicine* 10, no. 6 (2011): 1–8.

18. Bradford S. Weeks, "Cholesterol Drugs Tied to Birth Defects," *WeeksMD* (blog), January 21, 2008, http://weeksmd.com/2008/01/cholesterol-drugs-tied-to-birth-defects/.

NR4. Steer Clear of Harmful Protein

1. Elan D. Louis et al., "Elevated Blood Harmane (1-Methyl-9H-Pyrido[3,4-*B*] Indole) Concentrations in Essential Tremor," *Neurotoxicology* 29, no. 2 (2008): 294–300.
2. Ibid.
3. E. D. Louis et al., "Elevation of Blood Beta-Carboline Alkaloids in Essential Tremor," *Neurology* 59, no. 12 (2002): 1940–44.
4. F. Oz, G. Kaban, and M. Kaya, "Effects of Cooking Methods and Levels on Formation of Heterocyclic Aromatic Amines in Chicken and Fish with Oasis Extraction Method," *LWT—Food Science and Technology* 43, no. 9 (2010): 1345–50.
5. David Brown, "The Recipe for Disaster That Killed 80 and Left a £5bn Bill," *Telegraph*, October 27, 2000, http://www.telegraph.co.uk/news/uknews/1371964/The-recipe-for-disaster-that-killed-80-and-left-a-5bn-bill.html.
6. Joseph Mercola, "Why Did Russians Ban an Appliance Found in 90% of American Homes?" *Mercola* (blog), May 18, 2010, http://articles.mercola.com/sites/articles/archive/2010/05/18/microwave-hazards.aspx.
7. "Microwave Cooking and Nutrition," *Harvard Health Publications*, accessed May 19, 2016, http://www.health.harvard.edu/staying-healthy/microwave-cooking-and-nutrition.

NR5. Choose Carbs Carefully

1. Lydia A. Bazzano et al., "Effects of Low-Carbohydrate and Low-Fat Diets: A Randomized Trial," *Annals of Internal Medicine* 161, no. 5 (2014): 309–18, accessed September 18, 2015, doi:10.7326/M14-0180.
2. "Arsenic in Your Food: Our Findings Show a Real Need for Federal Standards for this Toxin," *Consumer Reports*, November 2011, http://www.

NATURAL REMEDIES FOR ESSENTIAL TREMOR

consumerreports.org/cro/magazine/2012/11/arsenic-in-your-food/index. htm.

3. Miriam E. Bocarsly et al., "High-Fructose Corn Syrup Causes Characteristics of Obesity in Rats: Increased Body Weight, Body Fat and Triglyceride Levels," *Pharmacology Biochemistry and Behavior* 97, no. 1 (2010): 101—106, accessed August 8, 2016, http://www.sciencedirect.com/science/article/pii/ S0091305710000614.

4. Meredith Melnick, "Studies: Why Diet Sodas Are No Benefit to Dieters," *Time*, June 29, 2011, http://healthland.time.com/2011/06/29/ studies-why-diet-sodas-are-no-boon-to-dieters/.

5. Guy Fagherazzi et al., "Consumption of Artificially and Sugar-Sweetened Beverages and Incident Type 2 Diabetes in the Etude Epidémiologique Auprès des Femmes de la Mutuelle Générale de l'Education Nationale–European Prospective Investigation into Cancer and Nutrition," *American Journal of Clinical Nutrition* 97, no. 3 (2013): 517–23, doi: 10.3945/ajcn.112.050997.

6. "Dr. Oz Investigates: Arsenic in Apple Juice," *The Dr. Oz Show*, accessed September 18, 2015, http://www.doctoroz.com/article/dr-oz-investigates-arsenic-apple-juice.

7. Joseph Mercola, "The Shocking Truth about Freshly Squeezed Orange Juice," *Mercola* (blog), August 16, 2011, http://articles.mercola.com/sites/ articles/archive/2011/08/16/dirty-little-secret-orange-juice-is-artificially-fla-vored-to-taste-like-oranges.aspx.

NR6. Reduce Stress

1. Amy Mattson, "Stress Hormone Linked to Short-Term Memory Loss as We Age," *Iowa Now*, June 17, 2014, http://now.uiowa.edu/2014/06/ stress-hormone-linked-short-term-memory-loss-we-age.

NR7. Get Quality Sleep

1. Alice Park, "The Power of Sleep: New Research Shows a Good Night's Rest Isn't a Luxury—It's Critical for Your Brain and for Your Health," *Time* 184, no. 11 (2014): 53–58.

2. "Can Sleep Affect Your Brain Size?" American Academy of Neurology, accessed November 2, 2014, https://www.aan.com/PressRoom/Home/PressRelease/1305.
3. Park, "The Power of Sleep."
4. G. Jean-Louis et al., "Melatonin Effects on Sleep, Mood, and Cognition in Elderly with Mild Cognitive Impairment," *Journal of Pineal Research* 25, no. 3 (1998):177–83.
5. Rensselaer Polytechnic Institute, "Light from Self-Luminous Tablet Computers Can Affect Evening Melatonin, Delaying Sleep," *Science Daily* (blog), August 27, 2012, https://www.sciencedaily.com/releases/2012/08/120827094211.htm.
6. Kristine Yaffe et al., "Sleep-Disordered Breathing, Hypoxia, and Risk of Mild Cognitive Impairment and Dementia in Older Women," *Journal of the American Medical Association* 306, no. 6 (2011): 613–19.

NR8. Balance Hormones

1. Zaldy S. Tan et al., "Thyroid Function and the Risk of Alzheimer Disease," *Archives of Internal Medicine* 168, no. 14 (2008): 1514–20.

NR9. Avoid Tremor-Inducing Drugs

1. "Health Concerns about Dairy Products," Physicians Committee for Responsible Medicine, accessed November 14, 2015, http://www.pcrm.org/health/diets/vegdiets/health-concerns-about-dairy-products.
2. D. M. Bhammar, S. S. Angadi, and G. A. Gaesser, "Effects of Fractionized and Continuous Exercise on 24-h Ambulatory Blood Pressure," PubMed, accessed November 6, 2015, http://www.ncbi.nlm.nih.gov/pubmed/22776874.

NR10. Catch Some Rays

1. Karl Michaëlsson et al., "Milk Intake and Risk of Mortality and Fractures in Women and Men: Cohort Studies," *British Medical Journal* 349, (2014), accessed August 11, 2016, http://www.bmj.com/content/349/bmj.g6015.

2. Mark J. Bolland et al., "Effect of Calcium Supplements on Risk of Myocardial Infarction and Cardiovascular Events: Meta-Analysis," *British Medical Journal* 341, (2010), accessed November 2, 2014, http://www.bmj.com/content/341/bmj.c3691.full.

NR11. Electromagnetic Fields

1. Devra Lee Davis, *Disconnect, The Truth About Cell Phone Radiation, What the Industry is Doing to Hide It, and How to Protect Your Family* (New York: Dutton, 2010).
2. Lennart Hardell et al., "Long-Term Use of Cellular Phones and Brain Tumors: Increased Risk Associated with Use for > or = 10 Years," *Occupational and Environmental Medicine* 64 (2007): 626–632.
3. Örjan Hallberg and L. Lloyd Morgan, "The Potential Impact of Mobile Phone Use on Trends in Brain and CNS Tumors," *Journal of Neurology and Neurophysiology* (2011), accessed November 2, 2014, http://www.omicsonline.org/2155-9562/2155-9562-S5-003.pdf.
4. Leif G. Salford et al., "Nerve Cell Damage in Mammalian Brain after Exposure to Microwaves from GSM Mobile Phones," *Environmental Health Perspectives* 111, no. 7 (2003): 881–83.
5. "Smart Meter Fires and Explosions," *EMF Safety Network*, accessed May 16, 2015, http://emfsafetynetwork.org/smart-meters/smart-meter-fires-and-explosions/.
6. Jennifer Abel, "Can You Become Allergic to Electrical Signals?: A Handful of People Settling in the Radio Quiet Zone Think So," Consumer Affairs, accessed April 5, 2014, http://www.consumeraffairs.com/news/can-you-become-allergic-to-electrical-signals-031014.html.
7. B. Blake Levitt and Henry Lai, "Biological Effects from Exposure to Electromagnetic Radiation Emitted by Cell Tower Base Stations and Other Antenna Arrays," *Environmental Reviews* 18 (2010): 36–395.
8. Örjan Hallberg and Olle Johansson, "Sleep on the Right Side—Get Cancer on the Left?" *Pathophysiology Journal* 17, no. 3 (2010): 157–160.

9. Gaétan Chevalier et al., "Earthing: Health Implications of Reconnecting the Human Body to the Earth's Surface Electrons," Hindawi, accessed June 30, 2015, http://www.hindawi.com/journals/jeph/2012/291541/.

NR12. Household Products

1. J. M. Gorell et al., "Parkinson's Disease with Exposure to Pesticides, Farming, Well Water, and Rural Living," *Neurology* 50, no. 5 (1998): 1346–50.
2. Cheryl Long, "Hazards of the World's Most Common Herbicide," *Mother Earth News* (blog), October/November 2005, http://www.motherearthnews.com/organic-gardening/hazards-of-the-worlds-most-common-herbicide.aspx#ixzz34MJMiAhT.
3. S. Costello et al., "Parkinson's Disease and Residential Exposure to Maneb and Paraquat from Agricultural Applications in the Central Valley of California," *American Journal of Epidemiology* 169, no. 8 (2009): 919–26.
4. "Methylene Chloride (Dichloromethane)," Environmental Protection Agency, accessed June 15, 2014, http://www.epa.gov/ttn/atw/hlthef/methylen.html.
5. "Tetrachloroethylene (Perchloroethylene)," Environmental Protection Agency, accessed June 15, 2014, http://www.epa.gov/ttnatw01/hlthef/tet-ethy.html.
6. "Toluene," Environmental Protection Agency, accessed June 15, 2014, http://www.epa.gov/ttn/atw/hlthef/toluene.html.
7. "1,3-Butadiene," OSHA, accessed June 15, 2014, https://www.osha.gov/SLTC/butadiene/index.html.
8. "1,3-Butadiene: Health Effects," OSHA, accessed June 15, 2014, https://www.osha.gov/SLTC/butadiene/healtheffects.html.

NR13. Toxic Metals

1. Midori Kato-Negishi and Masahiro Kawahara, "Link between Aluminum and the Pathogenesis of Alzheimer's Disease: The Integration of the Aluminum

and Amyloid Cascade Hypotheses," Hindawi, accessed June 15, 2014, http://www.hindawi.com/journals/ijad/2011/276393/.

2. George J. Brewer, "Copper Excess, Zinc Deficiency, and Cognition Loss in Alzheimer's Disease," *BioFactors* 38, no. 2 (2012): 107–13.

3. Erica Wickham, "Signs and Symptoms of Taking Too Much Iron," *Livestrong* (blog) August 16, 2013, http://www.livestrong.com/article/360738-signs-and-symptoms-of-taking-too-much-iron/#ixz-z2Ob2RMvVe.

4. E. D. Louis et al., "Association between Essential Tremor and Blood Lead Concentration," *Environmental Health Perspectives* 111, no. 14 (2003): 1707–11.

5. O. Dogu et al., "Elevated Blood Lead Concentrations of Essential Tremor: A Case-Control Study in Mersin, Turkey," *Environmental Health Perspectives* 115, no. 11 (2007): 1564–68.

NR14. Vaccinations

1. David Michael Augenstein, "New Study: Vaccinated Children Have 2 to 5 Times More Diseases and Disorders than Unvaccinated Children," *Health Impact News* (blog), October 10, 2011, http://healthimpactnews.com/2011/new-study-vaccinated-children-have-2-to-5-times-more-diseases-and-dis-orders-than-unvaccinated-children/.

2. Joseph Mercola, "Hepatitis B Vaccine: Refuse This Routine Procedure—Or Expose Your Baby's Brain to Severe Danger," *Mercola* (blog), November 3, 2011, http://articles.mercola.com/sites/articles/archive/2010/11/03/hepatitis-b-vaccines-at-birth.aspx.

3. "Judicial Watch Uncovers FDA Gardasil Records Detailing 26 New Reported Deaths," *Judicial Watch* (blog), October 19, 2011, http://www.judicialwatch.org/press-room/press-releases/judicial-watch-uncovers-fda-gardasil-records-detailing-26-new-reported-deaths/.

4. "Vaccine Excipient and Media Summary: Excipients Included in US Vaccines, by Vaccine," Centers for Disease Control and Prevention, accessed May 21, 2016, http://www.cdc.gov/vaccines/pubs/pink-book/downloads/appendices/B/excipient-table-2.pdf.

5. Jean Dodds, "A Pilot Study: 1/2 Dose Vaccines for Small Dogs," *Dr. Jean Dodd's Pet Health Resource* (blog), January 17, 2016, http://drjeandoddspethealthresource.tumblr.com/post/137503224896/half-dose-vaccine-small-dog-vaccine-study#.V4GXcKJ50x0.

NR15. Antioxidants

1. Steven D. Ehrlich, "Alpha-Lipoic Acid," University of Maryland Medical Center, accessed October 10, 2014, http://umm.edu/health/medical/altmed/supplement/alphalipoic-acid.

2. "Alpha-Lipoic Acid," *Drugs* (blog), 2009, accessed October 10, 2014, http://www.drugs.com/npp/alpha-lipoic-acid.html.

3. J. S. Park et al., "Astaxanthin Decreased Oxidative Stress and Inflammation and Enhanced Immune Response in Humans," *Medscape* (blog), accessed October 10, 2015, http://www.medscape.com/medline/abstract/20205737.

4. Steven D. Ehrlich, "Coenzyme Q10," University of Maryland Medical Center, accessed October 10, 2014, http://umm.edu/health/medical/altmed/supplement/coenzyme-q10#ixzz364ZQNmdw.

5. M. Dumont et al., "Coenzyme Q10 Decreases Amyloid Pathology and Improves Behavior in a Transgenic Mouse Model of Alzheimer's Disease," *Journal of Alzheimer's Disease* 27, no. 1 (2011): 211–23.

6. Stephen Sinatra, "Is Ubiquinol C0Q10 Better than Ubiqinone? Surprising Results from My Own Research," *Dr. Sinatra* (blog), May 21, 2016, http://www.drsinatra.com/is-ubuquinol-coq10-better-than-ubiquinone-surprising-results-from-my-own-research/.

7. Tze-Pin Ng, et al., "Curry Consumption and Cognitive Function in the Elderly," *American Journal of Epidemiology* (2006), accessed July 8, 2016, https://aje.oxfordjournals.org/content/164/9/898.full.

8. Dale Kiefer, "Novel Turmeric Compound Delivers Much More Curcumin to the Blood," *Life Extension Magazine*, October 2007, http://www.lifeextension.com/Magazine/2007/10/report_curcumin/Page-02.

9. M. Belviranli, "Curcumin Improves Spatial Memory and Decreases Oxidative Damage in Aged Female Rats," *Biogerontology* 14, no. 2 (2013): 187–96.

10. D. M. Townsend et al., "The Importance of Glutathione in Human Disease," *Biomedicine and Pharmacotherapy* 57, no. 3–4 (2003): 145–55.

11. Tak Yee Aw et al., "Oral Glutathione Increases Tissue Glutathione in Vivo," *Chemico-Biological Interactions* 80, no. 1 (1991): 89—97.

12. T.M. Hagen et al., "Bioavailability of Dietary Glutathione: Effect on Plasma Concentration", *The American Journal of Physiology* 259, no. 4 (1990): G524–G529.

NR16. B–Complex Vitamins

1. R. Clarke et al., "Low Vitamin B-12 Status and Risk of Cognitive Decline in Older Adults," *American Journal of Clinical Nutrition* 86, no. 5 (2007): 1384–91.

2. "Riboflavin: New Treatment for ET?" International Essential Tremor Foundation, accessed October 31, 2014, http://www.essentialtremor. org/research/research-in-the-news/research-news-archive-2011-10/ riboflavin/.

NR17. Choline

1. "Structural States of a Brain Receptor Revealed," National Institutes of Health, accessed April 25, 2015, http://www.nih.gov/researchmatters/ august2014/08252014receptor.htm.

2. "Essential Tremor: Choline," Beth Israel Deaconess Medical Center, accessed October 8, 2013, www.bidmc.org/YourHealth/Conditions-AZ/ Essential-tremor.aspx?ChunkID=21658.

3. Ammar Mubaidin et al., "Citicoline in the Treatment of Essential Tremor." *Journal of the Royal Medical Services* 18, no. 1 (2011): 20–25.

NR18. Magnesium

1. Carolyn Dean, *The Magnesium Miracle* (New York: Ballantine Books, 2007), xvii.
2. Roddy Scheer and Doug Moss, "Dirt Poor: Have Fruits and Vegetables Become Less Nutritious?" *Scientific American* (blog), April 27, 2011, http://www.scientificamerican.com/article/soil-depletion-and-nutrition-loss/.
3. H. G. Classen, "Magnesium Orotate—Experimental and Clinical Evidence," *Romanian Journal of Internal Medicine* 42, no. 3 (2004): 491–501.
4. Cell Press, "Magnesium Supplement Boosts Brain Power," *Science Daily* (blog), February 2, 2010, http://www.sciencedaily.com/releases/2010/01/100127121524.htm.

NR19. Neurotransmitters

1. Billie J. Sahley and Katherine M. Birkner, *Heal with Amino Acids and Nutrients: Survive Stress/Anxiety, Pain, Depression, & More without Drugs—What to Use and When* (San Antonio: Pain and Press Publications, 2011), 13.
2. Ibid., 81.
3. "Researchers Identify Likely Cause of Essential Tremor," *News-Medical* (blog) December 7, 2011, http://www.news-medical.net/news/20111207/Researchers-identify-likely-cause-of-essential-tremor.aspx.
4. Sahley and Birkner, *Heal with Amino Acids*, 45–46.
5. C. C. Streeter et al., "Yoga Asana Sessions Increase Brain GABA Levels: A Pilot Study," PubMed, accessed November 22, 2015, http://www.ncbi.nlm.nih.gov/pubmed/17532734.

NR20. Herbs That Calm

1. Richard Mabey et al., *The New Age Herbalist* (New York: Simon & Schuster, 1988), 49.

2. American Association for Cancer Research, "Hops Compound May Prevent Prostate Cancer." *Science Daily* (blog), December 10, 2009, www.sciencedaily.com/releases/2009/12/091208191954.htm.
3. James Bowe et al., "The Hop Phytoestrogen, 8-Prenylnaringenin, Reverses the Ovariectomy-Induced Rise in Skin Temperature in an Animal Model of Menopausal Hot Flushes," *Journal of Endocrinology* 191, no. 2 (2006): 399–405.
4. "Passionflower: MedlinePlus Supplements," MedlinePlus, accessed October 8, 2014, http://www.nlm.nih.gov/medlineplus/druginfo/natural/871.html.
5. Steven D. Ehrlich, "Passionflower," University of Maryland Medical Center, June 23, 2011, accessed October 8, 2014, http://umm.edu/health/medical/altmed/herb/passionflower.
6. G. Engels, "Skullcap," *HerbalGram: The Journal of the American Botanical Council* 83 (2009): 1–2.

NR21. Acupuncture

1. K. M. Sui and X. Li, "Clinical Observation on Acupuncture Combined with Medication for Treatment of Essential Tremor," PubMed, accessed October 7, 2012, http://www.ncbi.nlm.nih.gov/pubmed/20214065.

NR22. Chiropractic

1. T. A. Hubbard and J. D. Kane, "Chiropractic Management of Essential Tremor and Migraine: A Case Report," *Journal of Chiropractic Medicine* 11, no. 2 (2012): 121–6.

NR23. Homeopathy

1. L. C. Mourão et al., "Additional Effects of Homeopathy on Chronic Periodontitis: A 1-Year Follow-up Randomized Clinical Trial," *Complementary Therapies in Clinical Practice* 20, no. 3 (2014): 141–6.

2. L. C. Mourão et al., "Additional Benefits of Homeopathy in the Treatment of Chronic Periodontitis: A Randomized Clinical Trial," *Complementary Therapies in Clinical Practice* 19, no. 4 (2013): 246–50.
3. K. Boehm et al., "Homeopathy in the Treatment of Fibromyalgia: A Comprehensive Literature Review and Meta-analysis," *Complementary Therapies in Medicine* 22, no. 4 (2014): 732–42.
4. L. Grimaldi-Bensouda et al., "Management of Upper Respiratory Tract Infections by Different Medical Practices, including Homeopathy, and Consumption of Antibiotics in Primary Care: The EPI3 Cohort Study in France 2007–2008," National Center for Biotechnology Information, accessed July 25, 2014, http://www.ncbi.nlm.nih.gov/pmc/articles/PMC3960096/.
5. R. T. Mathie et al., "Outcomes from Homeopathic Prescribing in Veterinary Practice: A Prospective, Research-Targeted, Pilot Study," *Homeopathy* 96, no. 1 (2007): 27–34.
6. Ambika Wauters, *The Homeopathy Bible*, (New York: Sterling Publishing, 2007).
7. "Homeopathic Remedies," accessed May 30, 2016, http://www.abchomeopathy.com/r.php/.

NR24. Meditation

1. Colin Allen, "The Benefits of Meditation," *Psychology Today* (blog), April 1, 2003, http://www.psychologytoday.com/articles/200304/the-benefits-meditation.
2. "Meditation and Stress: Help for People with ET," International Essential Tremor Foundation, accessed July 25, 2014, http://essentialtremor.org/wp-content/uploads/2013/10/Meditation-and-stress-help-for-people-with-ET.pdf.

Appendix B. Importance of Good Oral Hygiene

1. Sally Fallon Morell, "Weston A. Price, DDS," Weston A. Price Foundation, accessed November 5, 2014, http://www.westonaprice.org/health-topics/weston-a-price-dds/.

2. S. Anki and D. Mirelman, "Antimicrobial Properties of Allicin from Garlic," National Center for Biotechnology Information, accessed September 1, 2016, http://www.ncbi.nlm.nih.gov/pubmed/10594976.

3. Bruce Fife, *Stop Alzheimer's Now! How to Prevent & Reverse Dementia, Parkinson's, ALS, Multiple Sclerosis & Other Neurodegenerative Disorders* (Colorado Springs: Piccadilly Books, 2011), 138.

Appendix C. Importance of Exercise

1. Dan Peterson, "Exercise Improves Old Brains," *Livescience* (blog), January 5, 2009, http://www.livescience.com/9604-exercise-improves-brains.html.

2. John J. Ratey, *Spark: The Revolutionary New Science of Exercise and the Brain* (New York: Little, Brown, 2008), 222.

3. "What I Need to Know About Physical Activity and Diabetes," National Diabetes Information Clearinghouse (NDIC), accessed October 27, 2014, http://diabetes.niddk.nih.gov/dm/pubs/physical_ez/.

4. Becky McCall, "Never Too Late to Start: Exercise Cuts CVD Death in Diabetes," *Medscape* (blog), November 25, 2013, http://www.medscape.com/viewarticle/814934.

5. Rob Stein, "Exercise Could Slow Aging of Body, Study Suggests," *Washington Post*, January 29, 2008, http://www.washingtonpost.com/wp-dyn/content/article/2008/01/28/AR2008012801873.html.

6. Weizmann Institute of Science, "Lifestyle Changes May Lengthen Telomeres, a Measure of Cell Aging," *ScienceDaily* (blog), September 17, 2014, http://www.sciencedaily.com/releases/2014/09/140917131634.htm.

7. Zosia Chustecka, "Exercise Reduces Risk of Colon Polyps, Resulting in Less Colon Cancer," *Medscape* (blog), accessed October 27, 2014, http://www.medscape.com/viewarticle/738649.

8. Alice Park, "Regular Exercise Can Help Lower Breast Cancer Risk," *Time*, June 25, 2012, http://healthland.time.com/2012/06/25/regular-exercise-may-lower-breast-cancer-risk/.

Appendix D. Inflammation and Chronic Disease

1. E. Cotti et al., "Association of Endodontic Infection with Detection of an Initial Lesion to the Cardiovascular System," *Journal of Endodontics* 37, no. 12 (2012): 1624–29.
2. "Alzheimer's Disease and Gum Health: Is There a Connection?" Fisher Center for Alzheimer's Research Foundation, accessed October 5, 2014, http://www.alzinfo.org/06/pym/feature/alzheimers-disease-and-gum-health-is-there-a-connection.
3. M. A. Wichmann et al., "Long-Term Systemic Inflammation and Cognitive Impairment in a Population-Based Cohort," *Journal of the American Geriatrics Society* 62, no. 9 (2014): 1683–91.

Made in the USA
Las Vegas, NV
10 May 2023

71852106R00155